# The Cannabis Oil Companion:
## A Comprehensive Beginners Guide to Hemp and Marijuana Oils

*By Douglas McCort*

## Notice of Rights

## Notice of Liability

## Medical Disclaimer

This book is not intended as a substitute for the medical advice of physicians. The reader should regularly consult a physician in matters relating to his/her health and particularly with respect to any symptoms that may require diagnosis or medical attention.

ISBN: 978-1530073245

Cover image ©istock.com
http://www.istockphoto.com/profile/gaspr13
Cover, book design and production by Douglas McCort
Published by 9500 Marketing
P.O. Box 55793
North Pole, AK 99705
Author Contact: 9500marketing@gmail.com

# Table of Contents

# Introduction

*I would like to try cannabis oil . . . but I don't know where to start.*
The above is one of the most common, recurring statements on my Facebook page dealing with the sale of legal hemp-based cannabis oils. Many folks have seen stories in the news and social media regarding cannabis oils or have had a loved one mention cannabis to them in reference to a particular treatment, but oftentimes, cannabis represents a brand new territory, especially for those who lack any type of background with cannabis use. Given the amount of misinformation many of us have grown up with regarding the use of cannabis or marijuana, this might elicit feelings of conflict among some, primarily for those who are now considering the plant from a whole new angle for the first time in their lives. For instance, instead of viewing cannabis negatively as a drug of abuse, these folks are slowly beginning to reconsider cannabis as perhaps being a beneficial tool for making a positive impact on health in a more natural way than what is currently being offered by pharmaceuticals.

With the advent of social media services (such as Facebook) over the last half-decade, anecdotal evidence of the benefits of cannabis is being shared by those located in more tolerant areas of the United States, such as Colorado and Washington. Certainly, it is popping up on people's radar with more and more frequency. People who had previously viewed cannabis in a largely negative light are doing double-takes when confronted head on with compelling testimonials from others regarding the therapeutic use of the plant across a seemingly wide spectrum of ailments.

This growing awareness is generating a sizable wave of people who are becoming interested in things like cannabis oils for the first time, and these folks are hopping online, looking to buy cannabis oil without really knowing what it is they are getting into, how to judge one oil from another, or even what type of oils, if any, are, in fact, legal for them to possess. This makes many of these folks easy marks for snake oil merchants that are looking to capitalize on the green rush, touting miracle cures for sale on common online marketplaces, such as Etsy.

As is the case with any product (and perhaps this would be especially true for any unregulated health supplement), the buyer must beware and exercise caution: unregulated often means untested. While there are fantastic products sold under the label of nutritional supplements, and there are many quality hemp-based cannabis oils that may be purchased legally online as nutraceuticals, there are also companies selling hemp-based cannabis oils that contain very little, if *any*, cannabinoids, or in some cases, containing amounts of the substance THC that would make the oil unlawful for purchase in much of the United States. It pays to be a bit cautious when purchasing these types of hemp-based cannabis oils online and to resist the urge to purchase the first product you come across. I will provide some tips in a later chapter of this book to aid you should you decide to look into the purchase of hemp-based cannabis oils online.

Not all cannabis oils are created equally, and in fact, just by the nature of every specific variety of *Cannabis* being somewhat unique in makeup, there is no way to currently weigh one against the other on equal merits. One might focus in on individual constituents, such as THC or CBD for some sort of metric, but the vast amount of substances involved in cannabis oils are unmeasured and have not been quantified adequately in most cases.

In light of the above, frequently, the initial questions I receive on social media boil down to: *What is the best oil to take for x ailment, and how do we get it?*

The basic concept I try to impart on folks right away is that whether it is marijuana oil or hemp oil (the difference between marijuana and hemp will be explained later), or cancer or insomnia, there is absolutely no *best* cannabis oil or strain of *Cannabis*. There is no miracle concoction that will magically cure illness in the terms that most people like to view things regarding pharmaceutical medications. One of the hard truths one must accept when working with cannabis is that what might work well for one person with one type of cannabis could be completely ineffective for another person attempting to treat the very same ailment.

To start with, let us approach these issues with the basic mindset that there is, in fact, no single *best* cannabis oil and expand on things a bit further from there with deeper explanations of the variables involved that make determining this assessment to be so difficult.

There are a multitude of reasons why one should not make blanket statements or assumptions about the efficacy of various cannabis oils across a range of conditions, and we will explore many of them during the course of this book. Fundamentally, it boils down to the extreme amount of variability in both the *Cannabis* plant and the human body.

All *Cannabis* plants are different, as are all human beings, with each one of us exhibiting unique chemistry and genetic diversity. When just these two basic facts combine, the result is a staggering amount of variation in the outcome when X plant is combined with Y person.

As many of the substances in *Cannabis* work in concert with our body's own endocannabinoid system, the underlying condition of that system has a great deal to do with how exogenous phytocannabinoids will, in turn, interact with a given person's unique chemistry. What works well for one patient might have little or no effect in another patient, and that might have little to do with the actual cannabis being used and more to do with the person's underlying endocannabinoid state or yet other factors. One plant or strain might work wonders, while dozens of other strains show no improvement at all—or could, in fact, even help exacerbate the condition being treated.

This scenario also helps to illustrate why modern medicine, which is built around the patentable isolation of compounds for pinpoint dosing and delivery, has largely failed to embrace cannabis in the face of the proliferation of manmade pharmaceuticals on a large scale during the last century. But prior to the spread of synthetic pharmaceuticals, cannabis was one of the most commonly used substances in the history of the American pharmacopoeia.

*Cannabis* plants present a witch's brew, so to speak, of substances: most of which are poorly understood and very hard, in fact, to even measure or quantify, currently. Most testing facilities that work with cannabis today are only able to test for a fraction of the hundreds of active substances found within the plants. This basic fact makes consistent dosing from patient to patient and from plant to plant an absolute nightmare under our traditional model of prescribing medication in the Western world.

Currently, most doctors prefer to prescribe isolated compounds that are carefully dispensed in regimented doses so that a consistent dose can be given with a fairly consistent effect in their patients. In fact, most Western doctors will not prescribe a medication that has no consistency from batch to batch. Additionally, pharmaceutical companies prefer to do research on isolates and novel delivery methods in order to secure patents on substances. A main reason for this is that corporations cannot patent a plant, so they invest large amounts of money into the research, development, and marketing of the resulting isolate(s). In fact, there are only two botanically based drugs approved for prescription use in the United States today, illustrating how rare, indeed, plant-based drugs are in Western medicine. In light of all of this, cannabis goes against our entire way of doing things as far as our current healthcare system goes.

Of course, as a species, we have been using many of these plants without knowing why they work for eons. Indigenous cultures have handed down wisdom regarding herbs and plants for centuries, and we still do not know why many of these plants work the way they do in the body: we just know that they do, in fact, work for many conditions. It was once commonplace to trust in plants and herbs before pharmaceutical companies started producing drugs based around many of the same substances found naturally in growing plants and touting them as superior versions of nature's design.

However, the manmade, so-called advances have come at a trade off. On one hand, we have ultra purified and/or modified substances sold by Big Pharma that are based on naturally occurring compounds or molecules. Pharmaceutical companies alter them slightly or modify the way in which they are delivered in the human body, and the company is then allowed to hold an exclusive patent on the substance for specific use for a given number of years. This allows doctors to know with confidence that what they give to patient X is the same as what they give to Y and that all patients given the drug can be expected to display a given range of outcomes and possible side effects. As a consumer, patients know that when they go to refill their prescription, they will be receiving the identical product each time. This balance provides a certain baseline of stability and consistency for all parties involved—for both doctors and patients, alike.

But to examine the other hand, what we are seeing after a century of use is that, in many cases, these ultra purified or synthetic versions of plant substances do not work as well when removed from the rest of the plants they were originally derived from. Actually, these synthetics can be quite dangerous when isolated, manipulated, and concentrated. The current state of high-powered, synthetic, prescription opiates that are killing people at far greater rates than the illicit natural opiates, such as heroin, illustrates this situation perfectly.

Cocaine or crack is another prime example. Native peoples in areas where coca grows wild have chewed the leaves of the plant for centuries. There are very few problems with its use at that level. But when man takes the base out of the coca leaves, chemically alters it, and further refines it into specific isolates, concentrated drugs such as cocaine and crack are the result as well as all of the associated harms that come from that unnatural increase in the levels of active substances naturally present and balanced in coca. What was once balanced and buffered by nature is turned into a potent poison when altered by man.

Many times, taking a substance out of nature's design and tweaking it is not such a good idea, after all. Nature, in most cases, it would seem, has already drawn up some very solid plans.

Our entire Western way of relying on isolated compounds is failing. In many cases, these pharmaceuticals are causing more disease than they are treating successfully. When a substance is removed from its naturally occurring matrix and isolated, the original design and balance, as it were, are lost. Whatever your concept of design in nature, be it Divine in origin or a product of Mother Nature, we have to stop to consider that the design of many plants do not need to be further improved upon by man. Man does not genetically modify fruits and vegetables to make them taste or perform better in the body. Corporations genetically modify crops to make them more economical to produce. Similar types of modifications are made to naturally occurring plant-based substances by the pharmaceutical industry, and then, they are remarketed to us as improved versions of Mother Nature's ancient designs. These are old tools that are being rebranded by corporations as new or better tools, and much of it boils down to little more than marketing tactics at the end of the day.

Focusing on the above in a practical analogy as it might apply to cannabis, if we take a complex dinner recipe, let us say chicken curry, and decide to omit everything but the main ingredient, we would be left with a boring, predictable meal of uninspiring chicken. It will fulfill the requirement for basic nourishment and protein, sure, but it will lack the intangibles . . . the magic . . . the things that make a great recipe stand out. It is the entourage of ingredients that leads to the final effect where any individual ingredient begins to pale when contrasted to the sum of each part, as opposed to when it is taken as a whole. I like to look at cannabis this way in as much as nature has already crafted the perfect recipes with all of the requisite parts in the many types of *Cannabis* plants.

The parts of the cannabis plant do not need to be isolated to make them better; we simply need to enhance our understanding of the ways in which whole-plant *Cannabis* interacts with the human body. It is a mistake on our part as a culture to attempt to simplify cannabis to the point of only discussing marijuana or hemp strains, or THC and CBD levels. By doing this, we run the risk of missing the much larger picture that cannabis has to offer as a whole. And it would be a mistake to assume that all cannabis preparations are the same and that all illness will respond in the same manner in every individual. This is truly personalized care, compliments of nature, as cannabis is not a mass produced manmade, artificial substance. It should be viewed as a plant and not as a medicine in the context that we have come to view medications over the last century. Cannabis is indeed a medicine, but one that strains the current definition of that term greatly as it has come to be used in our culture in terms of our current expectations with regard to prescription medications.

In an era when we like to fool ourselves into thinking we have some of life's fundamental mysteries cracked, cannabis offers up a riddle, wrapped in an enigma. Despite isolating many of the active compounds in cannabis some 50 years ago, we still, in fact, know very little about what these substances do in the human body. This is in part due to the legal climate surrounding the plant since the time of the Nixon administration and the creation of the War on Drugs in the 1970s. This climate has prevented any legitimate, funded research into the positive effects of cannabis use for a half century now.

Much of the data currently available regarding the therapeutic use of cannabis lies in the form of anecdotal reports from folks that have been utilizing it to varying degrees of success for the treatment of a wide range of conditions over the last 50 years. Very little information is based on science as the term typically applies to medicine. Cannabis takes us back to a time before pharmaceutical companies when we used to trust in the wisdom of plants and herbs.

Indigenous peoples across the planet have used healing plants and herbs for time immemorial. However, today, the United States, as a country, is one of the most reliant on manmade pharmaceuticals; yet, it enjoys a standard of health that consistently ranks well behind many nations of the world. Much of the illnesses faced are complicated and exacerbated by Big Pharma. As a culture, we have come to look to the treatment of symptoms with isolates when we should be looking to the root cause of our illnesses and treating them from that direction—from the foundation up, as it were. Think about it like this: It does no good to fix the leak in the roof if the foundation is already rotten; the building will ultimately collapse in spite of the roof repairs. Sure, the pesky leak is gone, but the root problem in the foundation remains to fester.

So when looking to consider cannabis for the first time, many folks will perhaps need to shake off a bit of this mentality that has permeated our culture so pervasively in the last century. The last 50-100 years have created a tradition in medicine of looking for the most well-marketed, synthetically produced pills meant to treat specific symptoms with little or no regard to the prevention of illness. And when all the best marketed pills fail or have unacceptable side effects, many people are now looking to cannabis oil as an alternative, but they are turning to the plant with this same mentality, assuming cannabis oil to be a consistent, easy thing to prescribe in a one-size-fits-all manner, similar to pills.

Quite simply, there is no *best* when looking at cannabis oils or medical marijuana. There is a tremendous amount of variation to consider when looking to try cannabis for a desired outcome. There are many types of cannabis oils, *Cannabis* strains, and cannabis compounds, so to try to reduce the concept of cannabis oil and describe it as an isolate, a singularity, is fruitless. This is symptomatic of our collective mindset toward medications in many respects. We are conditioned to a certain expectation in regard to medications, consistency, and the effects when taking said medications.

Choosing to use cannabis is a leap of faith. It requires faith and belief in the plant and its endless possibilities, and faith that what you are doing is right for you. Accept the fact now that there will always likely be more that you will not understand about cannabis than what you do understand, as far as how it works in our bodies, and just embrace that going forward. Even people like me, who have been looking at cannabis for 30 years now, are still constantly learning new things about it. We all have much to learn.

Folks coming from the recreational side of marijuana into the medicinal side are used to this leap into the unknown and the amount of uncertainty that naturally accompanies a typical cannabis transaction. The required leap of faith, in the medicinal sense, is much easier for people with this type of background to make. The fact that they might need to try many strains to find the one or ones that particularly favor their own unique bodies and chemistry is not a surprise to them. They already consider that to be part and parcel of cannabis culture similar to the way a wine aficionado would be aware of all the various intricacies involved with selecting a particular wine to accompany a particular meal.

For those coming into cannabis cold, however, this concept could be quite a shock. This leap of faith that is necessary with cannabis and the need for individual trial and error is foreign to most that have traditionally looked to their doctors for guidance on how to treat illness. Cannabis use is about empowering yourself to utilize a plant to manipulate your body's own endocannabinoid system in a natural way, and YOU will be the ultimate judge as far as efficacy goes. You can turn to others for suggestions and advice, sure, but at the end of the day, you will be the final judge to determine what works best for you and your own body.

This book has been written with the above concepts in mind. However, please note that although cannabis is a leap of faith in many respects, we can certainly educate ourselves about what we do know scientifically about the various differences in plants and substances that cannabis has to offer in order to better utilize it as a healing tool. By understanding some of the basic, individual elements of the *Cannabis* plant and cannabis extracts, we can begin to appreciate the larger picture as a whole as well as how these various elements work together to help explain the overall effects observed with cannabis as it relates back to individual illness.

This book will look primarily at the variances in cannabis, as the variance in individual illness would be far beyond the scope of this text, but the overall concepts can be applied to the treatment of any illness for which cannabis use is indicated. By understanding the parts, you will have a better understanding on how to apply it to your whole, individual picture. I cannot stress this enough: *Cannabis oil is an individual medicine.* It is not a lowest common denominator, take-a-pill-and-call-me-in-the-morning substance. If you keep that in mind, then you will be fine. Cannabis will lead the way: you just have to learn to listen to your body and instinct (rather than being told by someone else, such as a doctor) and be ready for a bit of trial and error with this plant until you find the variants that work well for you and your body.

This may prove difficult for some more than others, as there are significant legal hurdles to contend with in many parts of the world with regard to cannabis that may severely impact one's ability to be particularly choosy about the type of cannabis oils that they want to employ. But this equation is changing rapidly, with more and more U.S. states enacting medical marijuana programs and some having outright legalized the plant. As much of the world follows U.S. drug policy, other countries are also beginning to question the prohibition of cannabis on both medicinal and recreational levels. As well, cannabis oils are now being derived from hemp for the first time in history, and this opens up a new, legal source of cannabis oil for those living in the many countries that currently accept hemp imports. The picture with regard to cannabis is changing almost daily now, so if looking to cannabis as an option, it is more important than ever to be aware of the differences in the various types of cannabis oils being produced. It is my hope that this book will help you to that end.

# Chapter I

# What is *Cannabis*?

Let us start with that basic question, as it is important to understand what the word cannabis actually means as opposed to its connotation or how it can be misperceived in popular culture in the year 2015.

*Cannabis* refers to a group of flowering herbs indigenous to various tropical regions of the world as well as the Hindu-Kush areas of south central Asia. These annual plants range in size from small bushes to small trees of 20 feet or more and rely on open pollination for reproduction between the male and female individuals. While *Cannabis* plants will typically display a sex, one or the other, hermaphroditism can also be a common trait, especially in hybrid cultivars, where the plant produces both male and female reproductive parts on the flowers, allowing the plant to self pollinate. Hemaphroditism can be triggered by environmental stress or genetic predisposition.

In popular nomenclature, the term cannabis has come to be closely associated with the term marijuana in contrast to the term hemp, which has retained its own individual distinction in everyday use. The term *marihuana* (original spelling meant to racialize the term) itself was introduced at the time of the prohibition of cannabis in the United States in the 1930s in an effort to tie its use back to scapegoat immigrant Mexicans and black jazz musicians who had been the victims of salacious news reports of insane acts of violence while under the demonic influence of this supposed dread weed.

Prior to this, the plants were simply referred to by most as cannabis. The term *marihuana* was a direct result of the fear mongering and heavy propaganda campaign meant to shore up the case for the ultimate prohibition of the plants in 1937, and marijuana has since largely replaced the term cannabis in popular culture.

## Historical Use

*Cannabis* has a long history of both medicinal and recreational use with associations between humans and cannabis use dating back as far as 6000 BC when the seeds were used for food by the Chinese. Its first appearance in the Chinese pharmacopoeia, regarding its medicinal use, was some time around 2700 BC. The smoking of hashish (the dried sifted resins of the *Cannabis* plant) as a recreational substance was a commonplace practice in many cultures by the 1200s.

In the early Americas, hemp was grown extensively across the country and cannabis was used commonly in the American pharmacopoeia throughout the 1800s until its prohibition in 1937 in light of the Marijuana Tax Act. Today, cannabis is the most widely used illicit drug on Earth.

*Cannabis* plants are nontoxic with no known lethal dose in humans. The estimated lethal dose would be physically prohibitive to consume due to the vast quantities required to provide such an outcome. Please note that, while some plants in the *Cannabis* genus are considered to be psychoactive based on their content of THC and other psychoactive compounds, not all species or strains of *Cannabis* display this psychoactivity.

Drug species and strains of *Cannabis* are typically grown as seedless females, what is termed *Sinsemilla,* with the male plants being disposed of early in the growth cycle in order to maximize the production of flowers and resins within the female plants. Hemp varieties of *Cannabis*, on the other hand, are traditionally allowed to grow inter-sexed in fields to encourage the production of seeds and fiber. *Cannabis* plants can be grown outdoors in natural conditions or raised indoors under artificial lighting where all environmental factors can be closely monitored and controlled.

## Species Designation

Plants in the *Cannabis* genus are typically split into three species: *Cannabis indica*, *Cannabis sativa*, and *Cannabis ruderalis*. However, there is a newly discovered fourth variety, quite rare and native only to Australia, affectionately known as *bastard Cannabis* due to its unearthly appearance, similar to much of the life forms that have evolved remotely in Australia.

For much of recent history, the collective plants' genus has been described as *Cannabis sativa L.* There are further subspecies classifications or strain designations that have been made, but for all intents and purposes, the above descriptors of *C. indica*, *C. sativa*, and *C. ruderalis* are what are used to classify most *Cannabis* today, and for the purposes of this book, I will be using the term *sativa* to indicate the species rather than the genus.

Think of *Cannabis* as the umbrella that the other species are all under. All three species can be interbred easily, which seems to indicate they are, in fact, all closely related with variances that can be attributed to the various environments in which the plants evolved rather than actual differences in the plants themselves.

Please note that *C. ruderalis* is sometimes also referred to as hemp or Ditchweed in popular nomenclature but that it is not necessarily hemp by definition per se. I will elaborate more on the definition of hemp shortly. Also, *bastard Cannabis* will not be discussed further, as it is a very newly discovered branch of the *Cannabis* genus found only rarely in Australia, and it exhibits very few of the typical traits for which the rest of the *Cannabis* species is well known. Understand that *C. ruderalis* and *bastard Cannabis* both serve to illustrate that *Cannabis* plants themselves are found growing wild, naturally, across the far reaches of the globe, from Siberia to Australia, from arctic environments to arid deserts.

## Are All Cannabis Plants Marijuana?

No. Look at the term marijuana as the umbrella that governments put certain strains of *Cannabis* plants under. In that respect, most governments in the world make two distinctions to describe all varieties of *Cannabis* plants. They are deemed to be either marijuana or hemp plants under law: marijuana plants being grown for drug production and non-psychoactive hemp plants being cultivated for industrial uses.

Some countries, such as the United States, make no current distinction between hemp and marijuana. Under the Controlled Substances Act in the United States, hemp and marijuana are, for all intents and purposes, treated as the same plant. Hemp's shared stigma with marijuana also stems from concerns from law enforcement about illicit marijuana being hidden within fields of hemp with no way to readily identify the two apart from one another. This is enough of a reason to help keep hemp intrinsically linked to marijuana under the Controlled Substances Act, and therefore, illegal to cultivate within U.S. borders. But this situation is rapidly evolving with the implementation of the 2014 Farm Bill, which provided language for the first time that made a legal distinction between hemp and marijuana in the U.S., coupled with the fact that many individual U.S. states have already enacted their own laws providing their own legal distinction between hemp and marijuana strains. Additionally, many other countries already make this distinction and permit the industrial production of hemp under international standards for certified hemp growing. For instance, Canada recently removed restrictions on the cultivation of hemp and is now one of the largest suppliers for imported hemp into the U.S.

All species and strains of *Cannabis* are capable of producing the same phytocannabinoids, terpenes, and flavonoids—be it a marijuana plant or a hemp plant. As far as Mother Nature is concerned, they are all *Cannabis* plants. Through selective breeding over many decades, however, farmers have molded the *Cannabis* plants to suit both industrial uses—such as seed and fiber in the case of hemp strains as well as breeding them for higher THC content in the case of marijuana strains. It is through laws on marijuana that things become a bit trickier to understand as far as discussion of terminology.

In its simplest legal terms, a *Cannabis* plant is considered to be a marijuana plant under most international law if it exceeds .3% level by dry weight of THC concentration (THC is a specific cannabinoid tied to psychoactivity in some strains of *Cannabis*; we will be exploring THC a bit later). Conversely, a hemp plant is simply a *Cannabis* plant that has less than .3% THC by dry weight. THC at this level of concentration will provide no significant psychoactive effect. This criterion has to do with the international regulations and conventions regarding certified industrial hemp, which is grown legally across the globe for a multitude of uses. Marijuana plants, on the other hand, produced for recreational use with a concentration of THC over .3%, are almost universally outlawed across the planet.

## Confusion of Terms

These descriptions became foggy in the United States in the 1970s with the introduction of the Controlled Substances Act, which placed both hemp and marijuana into the same category under U.S. law. This is despite hemp having none of the psychoactive properties of marijuana due to its inherent lack of THC as well as despite the fact that hemp had been grown in the U.S. for centuries without any confusion between it and medical or recreational marijuana strains. Since THC is the metric used to describe the psychoactivity in *Cannabis* plants, THC levels become the legal line in the sand when describing whether the plant is a non-psychoactive hemp plant or a marijuana plant.

So to be clear, all marijuana plants are *Cannabis* plants and all hemp plants are *Cannabis* plants, but hemp is not, in fact, marijuana, as silly as that is to read!

This has led to much confusion over the years as to what these terms actually mean—be it hemp, marijuana, or cannabis—and has consequently led to a fair amount of misconceptions about the word hemp, in particular. Hemp has suffered the stigma of its seemingly unruly, often misunderstood, cousin for the better part of a century now, despite sharing none of marijuana's inherent psychoactive properties.

Currently, in mid-2015, in the United States, hemp is still considered to be the same as marijuana under the Controlled Substances Act (CSA). The 2104 Farm Bill provided legal precedent as far as providing distinction between hemp and marijuana for the first time in the U.S., but it did not remove hemp from the CSA descriptions of cannabis and marijuana. Pending legislation, H.R. 525, the Industrial Farming Act of 2015, will seek to sever this relationship between hemp and marijuana for good under the CSA definitions of cannabis. In the meantime, the 2014 Farm Bill has opened the door for some 19 states now to start pilot hemp projects tied to university research programs and state agricultural development programs. Many of these farms are producing female hemp grown explicitly for cannabinoid production, particularly cannabidiol (CBD) production.

Additionally, just this month of July in 2015, a gene has finally been identified that helps to distinguish between hemp and marijuana strains of *Cannabis*, further eroding the legal position in the United States that all *Cannabis* is the same under law.

In 2014, Kentucky became the first U.S. state to successfully import Drug Enforcement Agency (DEA) permitted certified hemp seed from overseas and thus became the first state to legally cultivate hemp under federal law in over 50 years. The DEA initially granted the permit for the seed to Kentucky, and then subsequently seized the stock when it arrived at U.S. borders, prompting Kentucky to sue the DEA for the return of the seed stock. Kentucky ultimately prevailed, setting the precedent for other states to now follow suit, with Tennessee being the latest to be granted permission from DEA to import certified hemp seed into the U.S.

As of mid-2015, hemp growth is poised to explode in the U.S. with all indications being that common sense has finally prevailed over ignorance with regard to this innocuous weed. Many of the early U.S. hemp farms are growing hemp for medicinal use and not for typical industrial uses, growing the plants in a completely different method that what has traditionally been done. The growth of this new hemp 2.0, if you will, is being done the way that marijuana plants have been traditionally grown: indoors, seedless, and with the focus being on flower and bud production rather than stalk and seed production. This marks the first time in history that hemp is being grown for cannabinoid production. This also represents an important turning point in the history of *Cannabis* cultivation.

There are many people, even within the cannabis community itself, that are unaware of this shift in the breeding and growing of *Cannabis* and hemp. They continue to cling to the old notion of what hemp plants have traditionally come to represent. However, their opinions are not mirrored by what is really going on with *Cannabis* breeding and production in the year 2015. This leads to much misinformation being spread online such as the notion that hemp oil is not cannabis oil or the notion that *only* marijuana oils have medicinal merit when this could not be further from the truth. ALL *Cannabis* plants are capable of producing the same cannabinoids when given the proper breeding and selection for traits. If it is possible to derive all of the components of *Cannabis* from legal hemp plants, other than THC, then this is a huge boon to people that do not need or want THC in their cannabis oils. Hemp strains offer some of the most exciting recessive genetics in the *Cannabis* gene pool right now, such as the genes for high CBD and CBG production. Because of this, hemp strains are being hybridized with marijuana strains to produce brand new plants with new characteristics or traits that have been lost to time. Hemp plants are just about to embark upon their second coming into the United States, and the plants will be grown, in many cases, much differently than the way they were grown 100 years ago in the U.S.

Now with some of the basic verbiage out of the way, and you

know what we are talking about in terms of the basic terminology with regard to cannabis, marijuana, and hemp, let us take a closer look at the different species of the *Cannabis* genus.

## Cannabis sativa

*Cannabis sativa* plants are indigenous to various tropical regions of the world and were found historically throughout South America and Asia as well as Africa. *C. sativa* plants grow similar to small trees, sometimes reaching up to 20 feet in height in the wild and typically display long, slender leaves with flowers that are described as *airy* in density. They require a very long flowering period being an equatorial variety, resulting in flowering times approaching 5 or 6 months, in some cases, to reach full maturity.

C. *sativa* is poorly suited to indoor growing due to these requirements, and it was not until the advent of indoor growing technology that *C. sativa* could be tamed, somewhat, and raised in a greenhouse environment.

C. *sativa* species have long been cherished for their clear, inspirational effects and energetic qualities, and in the broadest brush sense of the term, they tend to offer what users describe as an *up* type effect. Electric, energetic, and sometimes *ampy* and heart racing, this type of herb can elicit anxiety attacks and paranoia in users with low tolerance or those already prone to anxiety. Some strains, such as those native to Thailand and Malawi in Africa, in particular, are notorious for being borderline hallucinogenic for all but the most seasoned smokers with effects that have been described by some as simply terrifying with these strains representing some of the most extreme expressions in psychoactivity within the *Cannabis* genus.

Most users would say that *C. sativas* offer a *head* effect, meaning the effect is mostly felt in the mind rather than throughout the entire body and many users prefer the clear-headed enhancement that *C. sativas* elicit over versions of cannabis that display a more profound *body* effect. These strains are often sought by medical users for use during the day because of their active, productive nature, and then, these same patients might prefer a *C. indica* strain in the evening when somnolence is welcome. *C. sativas* can be useful with depression, fatigue, anxiety, pain, and PTSD (among many other uses).

Common recreational and medicinal pure *C. sativa* strains carry familiar names, such as Thai Stick, Haze, Durban Poison, Colombian, Oaxacan, Malawi, Panama Red, and Acapulco Gold.

## Cannabis indica

The *Cannabis indica* species of *Cannabis* are indigenous to the desert and mountains of the Hindu Kush region with some of the first known samples having been described in India in the late 1700s. In contrast to the treelike *C. sativa*, *C. indica* plants tend to grow short and squat with fat leaves, more like a bush or shrub, and have a much shorter flowering time of 6 to 8 weeks due to the harsh locations and short growing seasons from which these plants originate.

*C. indicas* have been a staple for centuries in many of the regions of the world famous for the production of hashish, such as Afghanistan and Morocco. Flowers of the *C. indica* species tend to be very dense and tight with little air in the buds. Where *C. sativas* in tropical locations form airy buds to prevent mold from occurring, *C. indica* plants from harsh desert and mountainous regions of Afghanistan and Pakistan form tight buds to help conserve water loss from evaporation.

Again, in the broadest sense of the classification, *C. indicas* are attributed with a *down* or more sedative effect. Effective with pain, nausea, insomnia, and anxiety, *C. indicas* represent the more mellow side of cannabis, typically. Increased appetite, followed by somnolence, are some of the well-known effects of good pure *C. indicas*, and these strains typically offer the closest thing to narcotic effects available in the *Cannabis* genus. Most users would say that *C. indicas* elicit a *body* effect, as the effects are felt throughout the body and muscles. Users often describe the effect as being *couch locked* (cannabis culture jargon in reference to one being so relaxed that they do not want to move from the couch/TV!). This could be a very welcome medicinal effect for a number of conditions where mild sedation is required or desired.

With the combination of a short stature and quick flowering time, these *C. indica* plants were perfect for indoor production when the art took off in Holland in the 1970s. When growing moved indoors, *C. indicas* were the natural fit and soon became the preferred variety for breeding in a greenhouse setting.

Some common, recreational, and medicinal pure *C. indica* varieties would include strains such as Afghani #1, Kush, Black Domina, Maple Leaf Indica, Original Northern Lights #1, Mazzar, and LA Confidential.

Author's note: I have stated in the simplest terms that *C. sativas* provide an *up* effect, while *C. indicas* provide a *down* effect. However, these are not hard truths, and in fact, since all *Cannabis* plants can produce the same cannabinoids, many strains of both *C. sativa* and *C. indica* display properties contrary to this basic *up* and *down* description of effect. That is to say, there are sleepy *C. sativas* and energetic *C. indicas*. Much of this is chalked up to the *entourage effect* of other cannabinoids, terpenes, and flavonoids, which we will explore in a future chapter. This is an important concept to start to think about now, though. It is very hard to put plants with literally hundreds of combinations of cannabinoids, terpenes, and flavonoids into the same boxes and have each fit neatly under one of three descriptions or species!

## Hybrids

When high output grow lights were invented and growers began moving indoors in places with liberal laws, such as was the case with

Holland and Alaska in the 1970s, breeders started working with landrace (naturally occurring *Cannabis* indigenous to specific regions of the globe) strains. In this, growers began to take longer flowering *C. sativas* and bred them with shorter flowering *C. indicas* to increase yields and reduce the flowering times while producing smaller, more compact plants in the process.

These hybrid plants represented the best qualities of both types of *Cannabis* within one plant, and as a result, hybrids have now become the most prevalent strains available worldwide. It has come to the point where the hybrid seeds have become so popular that they are now being grown in areas of the world where native peoples only grew local landrace strains, and the hybrids are now wiping out these ancient genetics 50 years later through the open pollination of indigenous stocks in the fields. However, there is a movement among certain growers and breeders to preserve these ancient genetics before they are lost for good, and there are breeders who specialize in only using and preserving these unique landrace strains.

What this means now for most is that unless you happen to live in a legal state or country where cannabis growing is tolerated, most marijuana available illicitly today is of hybrid descent with very few pure samples of either *C. sativa* or *C. indica* available.

Hemp hybrids have also been produced by growers adding various hemp genetics into the marijuana side of the gene pool, resulting in some very new and exciting medicinal strains, such as Charlotte's Web.

Some common hybrid recreational and medicinal strains would be as follows: Skunk, Northern Lights, Big Bud, Hash Plant, Jack Herrer, Cinderella 99, White Widow, Blueberry, Cheese, and AK 47.

## *Cannabis ruderalis*

The *Cannabis ruderalis* species of *Cannabis* are thought to have originated in the Siberian region of Russia and exhibit unique auto-flowering traits, whereas other *Cannabis* plants rely on the photoperiod and day/night cycle to trigger a flowering response. *C. ruderalis* plants grow small due to their auto-flowering nature, as the change to undergo flowering is triggered a few weeks into growth, regardless of photoperiod. These plants typically display very low levels of psychoactive THC while showing high levels of the cannabinoid CBD. Some industrial hemp strains that contain *C. ruderalis* genetics, such as Finola, are grown commercially in Finland, Scandinavia, and Canada, but all *C. ruderalis* is not considered to be hemp, per se.

*C. ruderalis* genetics have recently also been incorporated into newly developed auto-flowering hybrids bred from traditional marijuana strains over the last decade originating with a strain called Lowrider, which is a C. *ruderalis*/Northern Lights/Williams Wonder cross.

With the new emphasis on CBD over the last several years, *C. ruderalis* strains are being looked at for breeding potential, as they carry the recessive genetics for CBD production that have been lost from modern hybrids, while they are still low enough in THC concentrations to qualify for industrial hemp status under law. After being regarded as Ditchweed for the better part of a century, interest in *C. ruderalis* genetics is picking up in the last decade due to the unique recessive traits it brings to the cannabis gene pool.

Those are basically the primary ways that most *Cannabis* plants and species are described today, and for most folks, it boils down to simply *C. sativa* or *C. indica* and marijuana or hemp. *C. ruderalis* is a term that is only used by breeders with knowledge of the strains—most people involved with cannabis culture being blissfully unaware of its existence or significance.

Now that we know something about all of these basic descriptors and classifications, let us take a look at the basic extract that can be derived from the plants—what is commonly referred to as cannabis oil.

# Chapter 2

# What Is Cannabis Oil and How Does It Work?

Cannabis oil refers to any extract of the *Cannabis* plant whereby the active ingredients and resins of the plant are separated from the green plant material and stalks, and thereby further concentrated into a liquid or resin form. A solvent or fat of some type is typically used to accomplish this separation process and can either be removed from the oil prior to consumption or be ingested along with the cannabis extract, as is the case of edible solvents, such as fats or cooking oils.

The active ingredients of cannabis are contained within thousands and thousands of tiny resin glands known as trichomes, which cover most structures of the plant and, in particular, the surfaces of the female flower. These glands help to protect the plant from high intensity light rays and create a sticky surface to which pollen grains and insects adhere.

These resin glands are insoluble in water and must be dissolved into a solvent to liberate them from plant surfaces. Solvents used for this purpose can be simple cooking oils or butter, alcohols (such as ethanol and isopropyl), or even super critical $CO_2$ extraction can be used whereby super cooled $CO_2$ is forced through the plant material at high pressures, leaving behind a clean, solvent-free extract.

We will get into the various types of cannabis oils and the various types of extraction techniques in a later chapter, but for now, let us just establish what qualifies as a cannabis oil. The oil, or extract of the *Cannabis* plant, is a sum of the cannabinoids, terpenes, flavonoids, and other substances contained within the trichomes of the plant. Waxes, chlorophyll, and other plant resins might also be contained in extracts that have not been thoroughly filtered and refined as byproducts of the extraction process, sometimes lending the oils an almost black appearance that is actually a very dark green color when smeared onto a white piece of paper, which is due to the excessive chlorophyll content.

Oils can range from opaque green/black to translucent amber in coloration—the more transparent, the cleaner and purer the extract, typically. Consistency of high quality cannabis oil is much like a pinesap or very thick honey. The oil is extremely sticky due to the pure resin content and becomes highly viscous with the addition of heat. Cannabis oils, like most oils, are flammable and will take and keep a flame after a basic combustion temperature is reached.

Cannabis oil is insoluble in water, so in many cases, the pure extract is diluted with a carrier substance, such as olive oil or glycerin, to bind to the oil and promote bioavailability. Olive oil and coconut oil are considered to be among the best carrier agents for cannabinoids, as they are highly fat-soluble and absorb well within the body.

We will explore more in detail on how to most effectively take cannabis oils in a later chapter. For now, let us just get used to some of the basic terms used when discussing the components of a cannabis oil so that you can effectively begin to judge for yourself certain criteria when evaluating oil for use or purchase.

## Phytocannabinoids

Phytocannabinoids refer to a class of compounds found primarily within plants of the *Cannabis* genus, but they have also been identified within the following plants (many of which have historically also been prized as healing or healthful plants): echinacea, certain liverworts used traditionally in New Zealand and Tasmania, flax, the kava plant, and black truffles, just to name a few.

The most well-known phytocannabinoid is delta-9-Tetrahydrocannabinol, or THC for short, and this is considered to be thc primary psychoactive substance found within the *Cannabis* plant. THC was first isolated from cannabis in 1964 by Israeli scientist Dr. Raphael Mechoulam who then went on to further isolate many other subsequent cannabinoids from the *Cannabis* plant. To date, over 100 known cannabinoids have been described within *Cannabis* with the current count in mid 2015 standing at 111.

In the last several years, a great deal of focus has been put upon another phytocannabinoid named cannabidiol, or CBD, due to recent research and anecdotal evidence regarding its use. To date, science and medical communities mostly emphasize research on THC and CBD with regard to the cannabinoids found in *Cannabis* plants.

While the active substances in *Cannabis* were isolated and described for the first time decades ago in the 1960s, it was not until discoveries made around 1990 that we began to understand how these substances actually interacted with the human body. These discoveries led us to what we now know and recognize as the endocannabinoid system.

## The Endocannabinoid System

It had long been presumed that receptor sites could be found for cannabinoids in the human brain, which is based on the previous discovery of receptor sites for plant-based substances, such as opioids. However, it was not until the synthesis of a THC analog developed by Pfizer in the 80s that scientists were able to successfully radiologically trace the locations of the cannabinoid receptors in the brain . . . and what they found when these receptors were mapped is that there were more of these types of receptors present in the human body than any other known type of neurotransmitter receptor.

In the 1990s, the first examination of this was put forth by science, which began to describe what was to become known as the endocannabinoid system and has since been found to exist in all animal life on the planet. This internal system of neurotransmitters and receptors has now been found throughout the body and was finally able to be outlined following the discovery of first the CB1 receptor in 1990, which was followed up by the discovery of the CB2 receptor in 1993.

Dr. Raphael Mechoulam, the man who had first isolated THC and CBD in the 1960s, was again at the forefront of this work with his team in the 90s. In 1992, Mechoulam and his group described a neurotransmitter that occurred naturally in the body that bound to the CB1 receptor. They named this neurotransmitter anandamide (*ananda* is Sanskrit for *bliss*). Anandamide is essentially the body's own version of THC.

Think of this relationship between these receptor sites and neurotransmitters as that of a key and a lock, and only these select substances will fit the lock on the receptor, opening it and then allowing signals to pass back and forth.

In 1995, a second endocannabinoid, dubbed 2-AG, was also discovered that was shown to be able to bind to both the CB1 and CB2 receptor sites.

A unique quality of substances such as anandamide and select cannabinoids is that they are able to perform what is known as retrograde signaling, which allows these neurotransmitters to form feedback loops. These loops help to regulate activity and balance over neurological connections. It is through this retrograde signaling that these substances are able to calm excessive neural activity in various regions of the body. If certain areas are over-stimulated, this retrograde signaling balance can help to calm these regions by allowing the signal to move back and forth, as it were, relying on feedback from the system to balance the system. This is a unique quality of the endocannabinoids (such as anandamide) and certain phytocannabinoids found within *Cannabis* plants. This quality offers an important clue to the ways that cannabinoids interact within the bodies of all animals on earth and how cannabinoids can provide harmony and balance within the body.

## CB1 and CB2 Receptor Sites

CB1 receptor sites have been found primarily located in the brain, central nervous system, liver, kidney, and lungs, while the CB2 receptor sites are located primarily within the immune system and in blood stem cells as well as being found in peripheral nerve terminals. The greatest concentration of CB2 receptor sites seem to be on B-lymphocytes and white blood cells known as natural killer cells. These natural killer cells serve to mobilize rapid action from the immune system in response to tumor formation, among other things, rapidly promoting the onset of apoptosis (cell death) in viral infected cells. This could be one potential explanation for the some of the anti-tumor properties displayed by certain substances contained within *Cannabis* plants.

The functions of the endocannabinoids anandamide and 2-AG are implicated in a multitude of body processes, such as memory function, bone growth/restoration, pain sensation, appetite, gastric function, motor function, cardiovascular function, and mood, to name but a few.

The discovery of this internal cannabinoid system has led to a modern revelation in understanding key basic processes in the body and offer a glimpse into the substances our bodies produce that help carry and regulate these traffic signals to keep things running smoothly.

The fact that we have receptors in our body that key specifically for plant substances like opioids and cannabinoids is rather astounding if you think about it. It seems to point to a synergy that we have either left behind in our modern quest for the next greatest pharmaceutical or do not yet have a grasp on in terms of its implications in our everyday health. The keys to these locks in our body occur naturally in nature, so in much the same way that we now understand our that bodies produce our own morphine in the form of endorphins, we now have come to understand that our body produces our own cannabis in the form of the endocannabinoids anandamide and 2-AG.

If something goes wrong with one's own body's internal endocannabinoid balance, it stands to reason that phytocannabinoids that bind to the same receptor sites as our own naturally produced endocannabinoids would be able to supplement a deficiency or stimulate an up or down regulation of these sites. For instance, we know that certain tumors express CB1 and CB2 receptor sites and application of phytocannabinoid agonists to these receptor sites seem to show promise in both apoptosis (cell death) and metastasis (spread of cancer cells to other areas), among other functions. In conditions such as epilepsy, substances in cannabis are showing effectiveness by perhaps acting on the CB1 receptor.

In the body, these substances work as both agonists and antagonists depending upon the function involved and, in other words, could increase or decrease activity at the given receptor site. This again is a unique function of cannabinoids. The fact that cannabis seems to be so effective across such a wide range of conditions starts to make sense when you begin to understand how the CB1 and CB2 receptors play a role in our bodies' most basic functions.

The substances contained within *Cannabis* seem to be able to fortify deficiencies in our own endocannabinoid system, allowing us to dramatically impact the areas of our body that these endocannabinoid receptors are found concentrated within, such as the immune system and nervous system. These areas are often ones that modern pharmaceuticals have failed to be able to manipulate successfully or safely for that matter, as most Big Pharma products attempt to shoehorn their way into the body instead of harmoniously crossing the blood-brain barrier and docking with naturally occurring receptor sites. This is one of the reasons *Cannabis* seems to be so safe for use when contrasted with many pharmaceuticals.

The study of the endocannabinoid system remains in its infancy with new receptor sites still being identified and more insight being gleaned into how this system is implicated in many of the body's most basic functions. However, we are light years ahead of where we were before the identification of this system in terms of beginning to understand exactly how phytocannabinoids interact with our bodies and how they may be used to impact health and healing in the body in a natural way. The notion that *Cannabis* can be used medicinally is no longer speculation: we now know *exactly* why these substances have medicinal value when ingested and it is due to the interaction of these substances with the body's own endocannabinoid systems.

Now that we know where these phytocannabinoids actually bind in our bodies, let us take a deeper look at some of the more prevalent cannabinoids and other active substances contained within *Cannabis* plants.

# Chapter 3:

# Cannabinoids, Terpenes, and the Entourage Effect.

Cannabis is an extremely complex plant made up of over 100 identified cannabinoids, as many as 200 terpenes, and a number of flavonoids that all show levels of activity in the test tube and laboratory. We tend to focus mainly on THC when it comes to cannabis, and the other cannabinoids have laid in the background for the most part, overshadowed by the headline-grabbing sensationalism that accompanies THC reporting in the media . . . that is until the last few years with attention being shifted to CBD.

Some 111 cannabinoids have now been identified, but even testing for the vast majority of them is very difficult, let alone quantifying their various effects in the test tube or human body. Most of the labs that currently test *Cannabis* are not able to test for the vast majority of these substances, yet. Further complicating the issue is the fact that even among the labs that are able to test for a few of these substances, there is no standardized protocol within the *Cannabis* testing industry itself. This means that you can take a sample to one lab and get one set of readings for THC or CBD concentration and then submit your samples to another lab, getting an entirely different set of numbers. Many labs still utilize cheaper testing processes that rely on heat to liberate the compounds, which will lead to a process known as decarboxylation with cannabinoids whereby heat will change the substances from one variant to another, significantly skewing the ending results. So one must take all *Cannabis* test results with a grain of salt, and it is safer to compare results from one specific testing facility than to compare results taken from many labs at this point in time, as there is simply no consistency from lab to lab.

When a single cannabinoid is taken out of this complex plant matrix of substances, isolating it and synthesizing it in the lab, the ending substance does not seem to perform as well as the whole-plant extract. This has played out in the lab as well as in practice with substances like Marinol (a synthetic version of THC), which has been on the market for decades. Patients who have used both medical marijuana and Marinol universally report that the herbal version is far superior with many objecting to the side effects of the pure THC in the synthetic version.

This has led to the description of what is termed by many as the entourage effect whereby the full complement of active substances is what is thought to provide the overall effect of cannabis—not just the isolates. Substances such as terpenes also have a profound effect upon the efficacy of the various cannabinoids in the body. When considering cannabis oil, the tendency is to talk about the THC or CBD levels, but really, one must stop to take into account the entourage effect present in good, whole-plant cannabis extracts.

In order to better understand these substances, let us dive into some of the most well-known cannabinoids and terpenes along with some of their observed effects.

## THC (Delta-9-Tetrahydocannabinol)

THC is the most prevalent cannabinoid found in cannabis (primarily contained within strains currently classified as marijuana under law), so we will start our discussion of cannabinoids there. THC is the primary psychoactive substance found in marijuana and can be found in some of the highest concentrations of any other cannabinoid. As stated before, this chemical closely mimics the body's own anandamide and displays activity on the very same receptor sites.

THC effects that have been anecdotally observed or reported in lab testing via test tube or test animals have revealed efficacy in the following ways/areas:

1. Pain management
2. Nausea and antiemetic
3. Appetite stimulant
4. Antioxidant
5. Intraocular pressure reduction
6. Muscle spasm suppression
7. Psychotropic
8. Bronchodilator

THC is one of only a handful of specifically scheduled cannabinoids in the United States with the remainder being synthetic designer drugs. THC derived from marijuana has been given a Schedule I status in the U.S. with no accepted medicinal use, carrying a (supposed) high potential for abuse.

Ironically, this same Schedule I substance, THC, when patented and distributed by a major pharmaceutical company (under the trade name Marinol, for instance) is classified currently as a Schedule III drug. In fact, Marinol has proven to be so safe after being on the market for some 30 years now that it was down ranked to its current Schedule III status, originally having been ranked as a Schedule II substance.

Unfortunately, however, as previously mentioned, substances like Marinol do not work for most that have used it, and patients time and time again show a preference for plant-based THC. The side effects of pure, synthetic, unbuffered THC are not typically tolerated well by many of the patients that have used it when contrasted with whole-plant marijuana.

This THC molecule, consequently, is currently scheduled as both Schedule I and III under U.S. law. If produced by nature, it is Schedule I. If synthesized by a pharmaceutical company, on the other hand, it is Schedule III. One version, the one produced in the *Cannabis* plant naturally, according National Institute on Drug Abuse (NIDA) and similar organizations, will destroy the mind and induce psychosis, among other horrible side effects. The other, as a

Schedule III substance, is approved for medicinal use, is available by a prescription from a doctor, and has a safety record that pharmaceutical companies would envy. However, in fact, the herbal version of THC shows less side effects and greater efficacy than the synthetic version, yet it remains a Schedule I substance. This points out the absurdity involved with the scheduling of this substance under current U.S. law, wherein naturally occurring THC is deemed to have no medicinal use and carries a high potential for abuse; yet, a pharmaceutical company has been permitted to patent and sell a synthetic version of THC for three decades now under a much less restrictive schedule due in part to its impeccable safety record!

While THC is typically the metric by which cannabis potency is measured, a closer look reveals a bit more to the story. For instance, it is fairly common knowledge among growers and long time users who have had a chance to sample (as well as test to verify THC levels) many strains of marijuana that in many, if not all cases, the individual's favorite strains—the ones he/she feels are the most potent—are rarely the ones with the highest THC concentrations. This points again to the interplay with the other substances in cannabis as having a profound outcome on the effects of a substance like THC on our bodies. THC is but one of many metrics to describe psychoactive potency in cannabis, but it tends to get all of the attention in the media and medical community.

THC acts as a powerful antioxidant in the body, and in fact, the federal government actually holds a patent on cannabinoids functioning as antioxidants and a neuroprotectives. This patent was taken out in 1998; yet, we are still told that marijuana has no accepted medicinal use, and with its designation as a Schedule I drug, cannabis is subject to the most stringent research restrictions and penalties for possession and use.

Schedule I designation for all intents and purposes prevents any funded research from being done on the substance, as it has already been deemed as having no medicinal value. This presents an unfortunate catch-22. We hear the cry loud and clear: *We need to legalize cannabis!* But *We need more research!* is the patent response. But no research may be done with a Schedule I substance. The costs associated with working with a Schedule I drug make it prohibitive for all but the largest pockets to even consider. It is far easier to design a synthetic version that a company can secure a patent on and then make their investment back on, since a patent on a plant or natural substance cannot be secured by developers.

While THC plays a very important part in marijuana chemistry, it is hardly the be all and end all of cannabinoids, and there are several others of interest that we will explore.

## THC Extra: A Word on Cannabis Potency and Exposing the Myth of the New and Dangerous So-Called Superweed!

*Today's marijuana is not your grandfather's marijuana!!!* How many times have we heard this rhetoric about the nightmares of today's high THC cannabis? *The nightmare of Skunk!!!* cry the papers in the United Kingdom. But is there any actual truth to this? Have THC levels really risen this dramatically in the last 50 years? In a word: NO. The truth is far less salacious.

Media and government statistics would have you believe THC levels in marijuana have doubled, tripled, even quadrupled over the last 5 decades, but in fact, since all the modern cannabis available is the result of breeding with landrace strains (that have been growing wild for eons), we are still just dealing with the same old genetics that have always been available. We have not re-engineered the *Cannabis* plant. The same high potency plants from Thailand, Columbia, Mexico, and Afghanistan from the 60s are the parents of today's modern strains.

Most knowledgeable growers would say that at best, we have managed about a 5% increase in THC in high potency cultivars over 5 decades of breeding for THC levels. A plant can only be pushed so far: it will not produce 50% THC. High potency strains are around 20-25% THC and have been that way since the beginning. High THC strains today might even push 30%, but this appears to be about the ceiling as far as THC production goes, and there are not many strains pushing that. Most are still in the low 20% range.

Skunk (recently demonized by the media in the United Kingdom), for instance, is a well-known hybrid that literally smells like a road kill skunk. It is an old hybrid mix of the following landrace strains: Afghani, Acapulco Gold, and Colombian. Once Skunk was created, it was so well received that it was bred into just about everything that came after it.

A great deal of modern hybrids' genetics have Skunk genes in them. As such, much of today's so-called superweeds can be traced to the ancient landrace genetics that comprised the Skunk hybrid to begin with. These strains are nothing new. The only thing that has changed is you do not have to live in Afghanistan, Columbia, or Mexico to sample those strains anymore: you can get them on virtually any street corner in the world now due to the proliferation of Skunk genetics, in particular.

Clearly, the overall potency has not changed; rather, only the wider availability of obscure genetics from Thailand and other remote regions of the globe have changed. The overall average quality of what is typically available on the street has gone up, but we have not engineered a new worrisome superweed that does not behave like the cannabis of old.

The main thing that has changed in cannabis' genetics over the last 50 years as they relate to marijuana is the loss of cannabidiol or CBD genes. As CBD mitigates many of the symptoms of THC psychoactivity, this quality was bred selectively from marijuana plants in favor of higher THC levels.

Marijuana began to be cultivated indoors where environmental factors could be strictly controlled and plants grown to optimum harvest conditions. Traditionally, it been grown outdoors, allowed to go to seed, and then smuggled in gas tanks and the like into various areas of the globe. This new indoor production led to an increase in quality and diversity in the strains available via the black market.

The United States' government will cite seizure data and contrast it to high quality indoor grown cannabis, stating that the THC levels are going through the roof, but this is simply not the case, as the bulk of what has been seized is poor quality marijuana imported from Mexico and seized at the border. There are many areas of the U.S. that do not rely on imported marijuana to meet local need.

The levels of THC in high quality samples have not changed in 50 years. What was high then is still high now. Anything else is pure hyperbole.

Perhaps the most important thing that is often overlooked when discussing THC levels is that increased potency is largely meaningless as cannabis users famously titrate their usage—that is to say that if presented with stronger cannabis, users simply use less than they would with a weaker strain, which translates to the same ending dose of THC and cannabinoids.

The superweed is a myth propagated by the government, NIDA, etc. Any marijuana would be considered superweed when contrasted with the poor quality imported marijuana smuggled in from Mexico, which made up the bulk of United States' drug seizures for decades thereby skewing the government's potency statistics dramatically. There is absolutely nothing to fear here.

## THCa

THC begins its life cycle (as many cannabinoids do) in the form of CBG or cannabigerol. CBG is the precursor to most cannabinoids produced in the *Cannabis* plant. From CBG, THCa is formed, which represents the acidic form of THC. THCa is the most prevalent cannabinoid found within freshly harvested marijuana varieties of cannabis, accounting for as much as 30% of the plant by weight and, unlike THC, lacks any inherent psychoactivity.

It is only through what is known as decarboxylation (the removal of a carbon atom, releasing $CO_2$), which occurs through heating or slow curing of the plant material, that THCa is converted into psychoactive THC. This is why marijuana is traditionally first dried and then heated for consumption through burning or cooking.

There has been quite a bit of focus on THCa in the epilepsy community in particular over the last few years with many patients reporting positive results from incorporating levels of THCa into their largely CBD-based medicinal oils and tinctures. Some potential effects of THCa include:

1. Anti-inflammatory
2. Appetite stimulant
3. Sleep aid
4. Antispasmodic

## CBD (Cannabidiol)

Cannabidiol (CBD) can be one of the most prevalent cannabinoids contained within certain varieties of the *Cannabis* plant. CBD, in similar fashion to THC, is first present in the plant in the acidic form of CBDa and then must be decarboxylated to become fully active in the human body.

Cannabidiol serves as nature's antidote to THC in many ways, balancing and reversing some of the psychoactive effects of THC in the body and easing uncomfortable symptoms of anxiety and paranoia that might accompany high levels of THC in some users. As a result of this trait, CBD has been selected against by breeders in favor of THC in recreational drug strains, and as a consequence, there is very little CBD to be found today in most modern hybrids.

Unless you live in a state or country that sanctions medical marijuana and allows dispensaries to stock many varieties of specialized *Cannabis* strains, finding decent levels of CBD in street marijuana is very challenging today. Cannabidiol is found in much higher concentrations in naturally occurring landrace strains as well as hemp and *C. ruderalis* varieties. Since industrial hemp has been selectively bred to have low levels of THC for legal reasons and to meet international trade criteria, the CBD levels were left untouched, and today, the reservoir for these recessive cannabidiol genetics lie within the hemp and *C. ruderalis* strains of the plant.

There has been a recent surge of interest in CBD in the medical marijuana world, prompting many breeders to begin work on hybridizing drug strains of *Cannabis* with hemp or *C. ruderalis* genetics to create modern, high CBD yielding/low THC strains— some of which are now approaching 20% CBD (or higher) in concentration. This marks the first time that *Cannabis* has been bred and grown to produce a specific cannabinoid other than THC, as there was never an economic incentive to do so before the recent focus on CBD.

Charlotte's Web, developed by the Stanley Brothers out of Colorado, is perhaps the most well-known high CBD hybrid to have been bred thus far. Many of the current high CBD hybrids are descendants of a strain called Cannatonic first developed by Resin seeds, which was a blend of the strains MK-Ultra and G13 Haze. Some phenotypes of this strain showed very high CBD concentrations, but it was hit or miss as far as stability, and only some of the plants displayed the high CBD trait.

Breeders, such as CBD Crew, began to work on stabilizing hybrids in seed form that would reliably produce plants with a 1:1 or better THC to CBD ratio and have created many lines around old standby marijuana strains over the last several years.

Some of the more familiar high CBD strains found today are AC/DC, Harlequin, Dance Hall, Cannatonic, Avidekel, Sour Tsunami, and Charlotte's Web.

Cannabidiol can be extracted efficiently from both hemp and marijuana strains of *Cannabis*, and cannabidiol derived from imported industrial hemp base is currently legal in mid-2015 to be sold across the United States and many other countries that accept hemp imports. However, domestic farms growing hybrid hemp exclusively for CBD production are already underway in the U.S. in the form of various university pilot projects as well as in progressive states, such as Colorado and Kentucky, which are growing state-legal hemp within their respective borders under the provisions of the 2014 Farm Bill.

Since hemp is still considered to be marijuana under federal law, domestic hemp products are still hindered by this association making them difficult to place into interstate commerce currently. In the meantime, hemp is imported in tons from the United States' neighbors in Canada and Europe.

Cannabidiol is not a specifically scheduled substance in the U.S. Only when derived from a marijuana strain does CBD fall under the Controlled Substance Act (CSA). The only reference to CBD in the CSA has been verified to be an internal reference code and is not a specific listing as a controlled substance. If derived from an industrial hemp plant, CBD, as any other cannabinoid, is legal in the U.S. when contained within hemp finishing products and nutraceuticals via HIA vs. DEA 2004, which exempts the cannabinoids found within non-psychoactive strains of *Cannabis*, i.e., hemp, from DEA regulation.

CBD is nontoxic and non-psychoactive, and can be consumed safely in large doses.

Cannabidiol in its two forms have been observed to display some of the following potential effects in test tube and lab animal studies as well as anecdotal reporting:

## CBDa

1. Anti-inflammatory
2. Anti-tumor/inhibits cancer cell growth

## CBD

1. Anxiolytic, Anti-anxiety
2. Sedative
3. Antispasmodic
4. Anticonvulsant

5. Inhibitor of cancer cell growth
6. Antibacterial
7. Anti-inflammatory
8. Anti-diabetic
9. Promotes the growth and restoration of bone
10. Vasorelaxant
11. Anti-nausea/vomiting
12. Antioxidant

CBD does not have a strong attraction to either the CB1 or CB2 receptors, but it has been found to be able to interact with them at very low levels in spite of this lack of affinity. CBD also helps to regulate the flow of the endocannabinoids anandamide and 2-AG on those receptor sites. There is much to suggest that there is also a synergistic effect gained when CBD is used in conjunction with THC as far as activity across these receptors goes.

Cannabidiol, along with curcumin found in turmeric, are recognized to be the most potent anti-inflammatory substances known to man, and CBD also displays powerful antispasmodic properties. Additionally, when serving as an antioxidant, cannabidiol is superior to both vitamin C and E in effect.

CBD has come to prominence, in particular, recently in the treatment of certain cases of intractable epilepsy, such as Dravet syndrome, gaining much mainstream media coverage and exposure over the last few years with anecdotal case reports coming out of states like Colorado that have state-sanctioned medical marijuana programs and legalized access to cannabis. The development of the Charlotte's Web hybrid strain in conjunction with the experimental treatment of a young Dravet syndrome patient, Charlotte Figi, over the last several years has cast a national spotlight upon CBD and its potential use in the treatment of otherwise intractable cases of epilepsy. Some of these patients have dropped from several hundred seizures a day to as little as a few a month after the introduction of various CBD-rich cannabis oils derived from both marijuana and hemp strains.

Cannabidiol has shown promise in a host of conditions, and it is currently the cannabinoid getting the most attention and early research around the globe. For instance, Israel is pioneering the use of CBD as first line treatment for their soldiers suffering traumatic brain injuries in the field.

CBD might have potential applications in the following areas (among many others): epilepsy, cancer, insomnia, anxiety, diabetes, nausea and vomiting disorders, drug addiction, nicotine withdrawal, benzodiazepine weans, multiple sclerosis, schizophrenia, depression, Parkinson's, traumatic brain injury, Crohn's and inflammatory bowel disease, autism, fibromyalgia, COPD, asthma, and osteoporosis. Again, this list is not exhaustive.

## Cannabigerol (CBG)

Cannabigerol acts as the precursor in the formation of many of the other cannabinoids, including both THC and CBD. As a result of this, there is not a very high concentration of CBG left in the *Cannabis* plants at harvest, as most of the CBG has since been converted to other substances. Extractors are beginning to look at ways to retrieve more CBG efficiently.

CBG is typically found in higher concentrations in hemp species of *Cannabis*, in particular, where it is a recessive trait similar to CBD production.

CBG is active on both the CB1 and CB2 receptors as well as other receptors in the body, and it also functions as a GABA uptake inhibitor.

CBG has shown potential for the following in laboratory, animal, and anecdotal observation:

1. Antioxidant
2. Anti-inflammatory
3. Anti-anxiety
4. Antidepressant
5. Anti-tumor

6. Intraocular pressure reducer

7. Antibacterial

Cannabigerol is not a specifically scheduled substance in the United States.


## Tetrahydrocannabivarin (THCV)

THCV is mildly psychoactive, causes euphoria, and serves to block some of the function of THC in the body while seemingly enhancing other functions of THC. THCV occurs only in trace amounts in most *Cannabis* strains; however, *C. sativas* of African heritage yield some of the highest concentrations known. This enhancing effect upon THC and perceived potency can help explain why certain African *C. sativas* are regarded as some of the most powerful cannabis plants on Earth with extreme levels of psychoactivity.

Some potential effects of THCV shown in laboratory and anecdotal evidence are the following:

1. Anti-epileptic
2. Anticonvulsant
3. Bone growth promoter
4. Appetite suppressor
6. Blood sugar reducer
7. Pain reducer
8. Euphoriant
9. Blocks some of the effects of THC

THCV is not a specifically scheduled substance in the United States but may qualify as an analog due to its close resemblance to THC. This puts it in a grey area on it own, as THC analogs are specifically prohibited under the Controlled Substances Act.


## Cannabinol (CBN)

If marijuana is heated beyond 250 degrees Fahrenheit or allowed to grow or cure for extended periods of time, THC further degrades into CBN or cannabinol. Cannabis oil producers will sometimes let their oils cook longer to decrease psychoactivity from THC and increase sedative qualities in the oil for medicinal usage, while most recreational users find the effects of CBN to be heavy, muddy, and undesirable in any significant quantity.

Growers are able to judge the conversion from THC to CBN in the plant by watching the progress of the trichomes as the plant matures under a jeweler's loop or scope, which start to turn from milky white to amber as they begin to age and die off. For a more sedative effect, growers will let the plant develop a higher percentage of amber glands before harvesting the plant. For very potent strains of cannabis, this can help to temper the effects of the other cannabinoids, helping to lower anxiety and paranoia that might be an issue for some users.

Some observed effects of cannabinol in the lab and anecdotal observations are as follows:

1. Sleep aid
2. Pain relief
3. Anti-nausea
4. Antispasmodic
5. Sedative
6. Contributes a muddy or foggy mental effect to cannabis

Cannabinol is not a specifically scheduled substance in the United States but likely may qualify as a THC analog under the Analog Act.


## Cannabichromene (CBC)

Cannabichromene is typically the second most abundant cannabinoid found in cannabis. A recent study indicates that CBC shows the ability to aid with the creation of neurons in the brain thereby acting as a stimulus on the processes involved with the creation of new brain cells and connections, especially in older brains such as those found in adults. This may have profound implications in the future treatment of illnesses such as Alzheimer's. Chemicals such as CBC in cannabis seem to promote neurogenesis (the formation of new cells) and more efficient connections within the brain. This flies in the face of the commonly held misconception that cannabis causes brain damage. CBC is non-psychoactive and shows a number of beneficial properties in observations. These include the following:

1. Pain relief
2. Anti-fungal
3. Anti-inflammatory
4. Antidepressant
5. Bone growth promoter
6. Anticancer proliferative
7. Inhibits uptake of anandamide

Cannabichromene is not a specifically scheduled substance in the United States.

## Wrapping up Cannabinoids

These represent the primary cannabinoids that may be tested for by most cannabis labs and some of the activities that these substances exhibit in lab and test tube data. There are over 100 more cannabinoids that are not listed here, and we have much to learn about in terms of both readily identifying them via testing labs and beginning to quantify their effects in the laboratory and in observations. More and more cannabinoids are being discovered every year with six new ones having been added in 2015, so far.

As more focus is placed on the other cannabinoids in cannabis, growers in more tolerant states/countries are beginning to cater to these other substances when breeding, increasing the diversity of cannabinoids available in over the counter offerings. While it can still be hard to find out if a particular strain of *Cannabis* has decent levels of CBC in it in most parts of the country, for someone in Washington or Colorado, this type of data, in many cases, is being offered at the local dispensary or retail outlet. In turn, this can give consumers much more flexibility when choosing strains for therapeutic use if they are aware of these other cannabinoids and the actions that they have within the body. Additionally, many websites online offer cannabinoid profiles of many common strains, which can help get an individual in the ballpark of which strain might work best for him/her when evaluating options. Legal hemp-based cannabis oils also offer access to many of these cannabinoids, such as CBC, CBD, CBDa, and CBN.

There is another primary group of active substances that play a significant role in the efficacy of cannabis oils, and they are what are collectively known as the terpenes and terpenoids. Let us take a look at those next!

## Terpenes

Another important constituent of cannabis oil that must be accounted for in terms of assessing medicinal activity are the important roles that terpenes and terpenoids play in the overall entourage effect that cannabis provides. Terpenes provide a synergistic effect in concert with the cannabinoids to potentiate the activity of those substances to a level of efficacy that is lacking when consumed as individual elements.

There are slight differences between terpenes and terpenoids, but for the remainder of the book, we will use the term terpene synonymously.

In contrast to cannabinoids, terpenes are quite familiar to all of us, regardless of previous exposure to cannabis use. Terpenes are some of the most recognized substances found in plants and are the chemicals that lend them their pungent and/or distinct aromas. Since the primary secretions in *Cannabis* plants are the resin glands or trichomes, it should come as no surprise that these plants are rich in terpene content, as terpenes are one of the primary building blocks of plant resins.

Perhaps the most familiar example of this would be the relationship of pine resins and turpentine, from which the term terpene originates.  Turpentine is a blend of the terpenes alpha- and beta-pinene, terpinolene, camphene, dipentene, and carene that are derived from the extracted resins of trees in the pine family.  Alpha-pinene is the most common terpene in nature and is one of the primary terpenes found in *Cannabis* as well.

Terpenes are large constituents of essential oils and as such are used heavily as fragrances in the perfume industry as well as finding attention in the alternative medicinal community via aromatherapy blends and tinctures.

These substances are used extensively for creating flavorings in the packaged food industry and are the chemicals that create many of our favorite plant-based odors (from citrus to fruit and from piney to earthy) to the not-so-favorite odor of rotten flesh.  The vast range of aromas that terpenes present make them a fascinating subject.

*Cannabis* plants can elicit a dynamic blend of fragrances and odors that run the range of every scent imaginable.  If there is a fruit, there is likely a corresponding *Cannabis* strain that smells like it with common scents/flavors being lemon, grapefruit, blueberry, cherry, strawberry, and pineapple.  There are *Cannabis* plants that smell like a road killed skunk, plants that smell like diesel fuel, and there are plants that smell like exotic incense.  All of these qualities are traced back to the individual terpene blends contained within each individual strain of *Cannabis*.

These very traits are what make up the some of the most desirable qualities in cannabis.  They are the subtle nuances from plant to plant that create personal favorites based on taste and smell, while providing subtle differences in effects from strain to strain.

When the 111 cannabinoids combine with the several dozen major and minor terpenes found within cannabis, the possible outcomes become truly staggering.  Not all *Cannabis* plants will produce the same terpenes or concentrations of cannabinoids.  One can literally go through dozens of strains in order to start to pinpoint what is most effective for them in terms of both cannabinoid and terpene composition.  Much of this data is very hard to come by via laboratory testing at the moment, though, so it becomes even more difficult to quantify these variables.

For this reason, the use of *Cannabis* can be largely a trial and error process with some strains outperforming others for certain conditions. And even within individual strains, there are tremendous variations in genetic expressions—even two plants of the same strain can display differing ratios of cannabinoids and terpenes.

Terpenes play a vital role in cannabis chemistry, and because of this, they should be taken into account when evaluating different strains or oils.  All strains and oils will have different terpene compositions.  If one is familiar with the concept of terpenes, he/she can begin to glean a deeper understanding about why certain strains or oils are more effective for him/her than others and use this information to hone in on specific terpene blends or spikes.

Again, information on terpene composition is still fairly young in terms of availability, but there are labs in legal states in the United States that are pushing this technology and allowing for the quantification of this data on a large scale. Also, there are breeders in Europe that have their strains tested for terpene composition, so there are online resources to find more of this detailed information on specific websites, like Leafly.com, for instance, that are starting to accumulate a nice set of data on many strains in terms of both terpene and cannabinoid profiles.

While there are too many terpenes found in *Cannabis* (at well over 100) to list, we will take a short look at some of the more prevalent ones as well as some of the ones with the most interesting medicinal activities. Unlike cannabinoids that are hampered by a Schedule I classification, individual terpenes have been studied extensively as the same terpenes found in *Cannabis* can be found within many other common plant species.

Some of the more common terpenes found within the *Cannabis* plant are as follows:

## A-Pinene

This is the most abundant terpene found in nature. Found in sage and pine trees, it is responsible for the piney smell in *Cannabis* and also serves as a powerful insect repellent. It can have the following effects on the body:

1. Bronchodilator
2. Anti-inflammatory
3. Pain relief
4. Antioxidant
5. Anticancer proliferative

## d-Limonene

This is the common citrus odor. It is found in citrus fruit, especially in the rinds, and in many lemon or citrus scented varieties of *Cannabis*. It is used as both a solvent and a cleaning agent in industrial applications, and can be used as a solvent for cannabis oil extraction as well. It has the following properties:

1. Antifungal
2. Relieves gastrointestinal reflux and heartburn
3. Antimicrobial
4. Anti-tumor
5. Antidepressant
6. Anti-anxiety
7. Increases bioavailability of other terpenes and chemicals in the body

## Myrcene

This terpene is found in mangoes, hops, bay leaves, thyme, and parsley (among many other common herbs and foods). Myrcene is one of the most important terpenes in terms of impacting the potency of cannabis and aiding in the efficacy of many of the other substances.    One can improve the absorption and potency of cannabis by simply consuming any of the above foods an hour or so prior to consuming cannabis.   Myrcene can exhibit the following properties in the body:

1.    Increases the effects of cannabis, a major player in the couchlock effect and increases the speed of onset of cannbinoids in the body.

2.    Increases the saturation level at the CB1 receptor, allowing for more cannabinoid uptake

3.    Allows for more efficient travel of various chemicals across the blood-brain barrier.

4.  Sedative

5.  Anti-inflammatory

6.  Pain reliever

7.  Anti-tumor

8.  Antispasmodic

9.  Muscle relaxant

## Linalool

This terpene has a floral, spicy odor.  Its pleasing smell is found in a great many fragrances used in personal cleansing products today.  It is found in cinnamon, mint, rosewood, citrus, lavender, and birch and can display the following effects in the body:

1.  Antipsychotic

2.  Anti-anxiety

3.  Antiepileptic

4.  Sleep aid

5.  Pain relief

## ß-Caryophyllene

This terpene has a spicy fragrance.  It is found commonly in pepper, cloves, basil, oregano, and hops.  Caryophyllene has the unique distinction of being a terpene with a known affinity for the CB2 receptor, making it very similar to a cannabinoid in terms of action in this sense. Caryophyllene is also an FDA approved additive in foods and is commonly consumed. As a side note, drug dogs are trained to detect caryophyllene as THC has no distinct odor for them to hone in on! The effects are as follows:

1. Anti-inflammatory
2. Antibacterial
3. Antifungal
4. Neuroprotective
5. Anxiolytic
6. Gastroprotectant

## Humulene

This terpene exhibits a hoppy fragrance. It is found in hops, coriander, sage, ginger, and ginseng with the following effects:

1. Anti-inflammatory
2. Appetite suppressant
3. Anti-tumor
4. Antibacterial

## Eucalyptol

This terpene has a spicy aroma. It is found in sage, basil, bay leaves, rosemary, and eucalyptus oil. It has the following properties:

1. Pain relief
2. Passes blood-brain barrier easily
3. Cough suppressant
4. Toxic in large doses

There are many other major and minor terpenes found in *Cannabis* plants, but those listed above are some of the more prevalent with the terpenes myrcene and d-Limonene having a particularly interesting role in cannabis chemistry due to their enhancing effects on the other substances. Many other common medicinal plants contain the very same terpenes as *Cannabis* plants as you can see from the lists of familiar herbs and plants above. It is not a coincidence that these other plants have also been used traditionally for centuries for healing purposes by many cultures. Terpenes help to explain many of the healing properties that these particular plants, including *Cannabis*, exhibit.

Now that we have a solid idea of what the major constituents of *Cannabis* plants are, let us examine how we can further apply this information as it relates to the broader topic of the use of cannabis oils.

# Chapter 4

# Cannabis Oils and Specific Illness: Treatment and Dosage Information

*Cannabis oils cured my _____ !!!*
When I see this statement, the next question that comes immediately to mind is, *What Cannabis strain was being used? C. indica, C. sativa, hybrid, hemp, high CBD, high THC . . . can this person be more specific?*

Cannabis or cannabis oil cures *such and such* is a blanket statement and one that can be misleading due to the sheer amount of variation displayed from person to person as well as the variation in various plants in the *Cannabis* genus, as we covered in the sections on cannabinoids and terpenes. It is vitally important to keep this in perspective when looking at things like cannabis oils. Cannabis use is trial and error. Everyone responds differently and each plant is different. This is one reason cannabis is not embraced by modern medicine at this time. Furthermore, it can be unpredictable and many of its properties are not understood yet by science.

Let us examine a couple of cases to illustrate the point.

Personally, I suffer from a condition called cyclical vomiting syndrome (CVS) or abdominal migraine. As a result of this, I am part of an online support group of fellow patients that all share information with one another about our illness and get support. One member, who had been able to experiment with dozens and dozens of strains of marijuana on his wife's condition reported ONE strain, of all of them, that would shut down an attack immediately. The others were ineffective, mildly effective, or selectively effective. Only ONE proved to have the best combination of cannabinoids for her.

In this particular case, this man's wife could have tried 10 different strains or oils and found none of them helped, leading his wife to declare, *Cannabis does not work for me*. If she, however, got lucky enough to find the one strain that helped amongst those 10 strains, she would then be likely to declare, *Cannabis oil is a cure*. It is important not to lose sight of this when hearing that cannabis does not work and/or hearing of miraculous recoveries or cures in regard to cannabis or cannabis oils.

Important questions to consider when discussing cannabis and its medicinal applications: What strain(s) of *Cannabis* was (were) used? Cannabis is not a reference to one standardized thing. What was the cannabinoid and terpene profile if available? What was the method of administration? What was the dose and for how long? These are all important questions, and in many cases, these details will be lacking, unfortunately.

As another example, in Colorado, there are scores of cases reported on in social media by families utilizing various cannabis oils to treat their children with sometimes otherwise intractable variants of epilepsy. Many of these families start with a high CBD/low THC hemp strain called Charlotte's Web. In some of these cases, Charlotte's Web has seemingly almost eradicated the seizure activity. Other children are not so lucky with Charlotte's Web, but have found effectiveness from oils derived from another local high CBD strain known as Haley's Hope.

Still other children are not responding to those base oils, but their families are having luck adding more THC or THCa into the CBD oils/tinctures, while still other children seem to get worse with any kind of cannabis altogether (often with the other conventionally prescribed drugs making the picture somewhat muddy as to what is causing a negative reaction). What we can glean from this is that every case is different and that there is no one-size-fits-all approach. We can say broadly that cannabis and high CBD *Cannabis* strains seem to have substantial antiepileptic potential, but we are not there, yet, in terms of assessing the supporting cast of cannabinoids and terpenes involved in order to maximize that benefit for any one, specific case.  We are still just using trial and error as well as watching what others are reporting, trying to draw associations.

Due to this situation, social media has become a huge reservoir of current anecdotal information that is now rapidly outpacing the last 50 years of stagnation in terms of research into the effects of cannabis.  If you want to see what is going on with people that are actually using cannabis to treat illness, social media is where you need to be looking.  It is hard to argue with testimonials from folks that are not selling anything: they are merely sharing their struggles and stories.  This is leading to a vast upheaval in terms of our general perception of cannabis being thought of as an agent of destruction rather than an angel of healing.

It is currently very hard to look to lab verified data due to the fact that almost all lab testing is done with synthetic isolations of these substances, as the whole-plant extract is a Schedule I substance and cannot be researched.  However, the isolates pale in comparison in terms of efficacy in many cases due to the entourage effect of the other supporting substances, which give cannabis its overall synergistic effects.

If you decide to look at cannabis or cannabis oils for therapeutic use, it is really quite important to become familiar with the various chemicals so that you can at least begin to attempt to hone in on strains that are more likely to help with whatever it is you are seeking to use them for.  This can also help keep you from having a bad experience when using full strength cannabis oils with THC in them, for instance.

A practical analysis of the above illustrations results in the following line of thought: A *Cannabis* strain that is rich in antitumor compounds might not be the preferred *Cannabis* strain to use for epilepsy.  A *Cannabis* strain that is stimulant in nature would not be one that would be effective in the treatment of insomnia.  A *Cannabis* strain that provokes anxiety would not the one to give to someone with panic attacks.  What this begins to illustrate is that, again, there is no one-size-fits-all when it comes to cannabis use.

## The 1:1 Ratio

There is a growing awareness regarding the efficacy of what has come to be known as the 1:1 ratio, describing a one-to-one ratio of THC to CBD. Sometimes this is also referred to as the golden ratio. A British pharmaceutical company by the name of GW Pharmaceuticals pioneered a 1:1 whole-plant extract, dubbed Sativex, which started development around 2003 and has since been approved for use in many countries for the treatment of multiple sclerosis, specifically. This drug is based on the 1:1 theory that had shown some promise prior to this product's development. Sativex has since been shown to be highly effective. It is a whole-plant cannabis product rather than being a synthetic derivative of a cannabis isolate. GW Pharmaceuticals is the only large pharmaceutical company currently doing research and development with whole-plant cannabis.

This one-to-one ratio is thought to potentiate the effects of both THC and CBD in the body along with the other cannabinoids. In fact, many *Cannabis* plants exhibited this natural balance in chemistry prior to extensive hybridization by man. For instance, medicinal tinctures used to contain much more CBD in the old days by virtue of the plants at the time being more balanced in composition.

While today presents a fractured *Cannabis* plant in some aspects with marijuana plants having very little CBD in them and hemp plants having very little THC in them, hybrids are being bred right now to cater to this desire for a 1:1 THC/CBD ratio. Until the widespread availability of these new strains comes about, there is compelling reason to consider using both types of cannabis oils if attempting to see if cannabis helps or not. This can be a way to essentially create your own 1-to-1 ratio oils with high THC marijuana oil supplemented by high CBD hemp oil.

Below are some of the conditions I have seen compelling anecdotal and/or scientific data published in some fashion, supporting the activity of some form of cannabis as being helpful:

Epilepsy, cancer, PTSD, Crohn's disease, irritable bowel syndrome, cyclical vomiting syndrome, diabetes, glaucoma, osteoporosis, social anxiety disorder, autism, fibromyalgia, nausea and vomiting, depression, Lou Gehrig's disease, COPD/asthma/emphysema, arthritis, chronic pain, neuropathy, AIDS, Alzheimer's, dementia, schizophrenia, ADHD, psoriasis, plantar warts, lesions, burns, multiple sclerosis, loss of appetite/wasting syndrome, anorexia, migraine, menstrual cramps, traumatic brain injury, colitis, hypertension, phantom limb pain, Tourette's syndrome, gastritis, agoraphobia, insomnia, gout, hepatitis C, impotence, Lyme disease, lymphoma, chronic fatigue syndrome, opiate dependence, seizures, sleep disorders . . . and the list goes on.

The list of illness and conditions that some form of cannabis is able to influence in one way or another seems almost too good to be true when you stare at it. And the conditions listed above are just some of the most well-known that have been associated with some sort of beneficial reaction to cannabis therapy. But when you consider the way that cannabis works in relation to how your own body's endocannabinoid system functions in the management of so many basic processes internally, it starts to make sense why this might be so as well as why the substances in cannabis could potentially be some of the most beneficial in nature for us to consume as a way of naturally restoring and balancing our bodies. Vitamin Weed, if you will.

## Dosing

In terms of dosing with cannabis oils, or any marijuana product—be it an edible or dry herb—there is again no set in stone approach or standardized protocol. You will have to experiment to find your own thresholds of desired activity. The one golden rule with cannabis, especially for anything containing THC, is to start out low and slow. If you have no background with cannabis and are just beginning its use for medicinal purposes, you will want to start very slowly to let your body build up a low tolerance level over a couple weeks' time. As you feel comfortable with the effects, you can slowly begin to increase dosage, as needed. This is all the more important when using concentrated oils or extracts that could have a potent psychoactive effect if taken in too large a dose.

This really comes into play a bit more with oral dosing, as smoking dry cannabis or vaporizing has the distinct advantage of making it rather easy to titrate dosage. That is to say, the effects are felt nearly instantly, making it easier to gauge whether you need more or need to stop right there. Taking an oral dose is much more of a commitment, and it will take an hour or more to take effect, but once it does, it could be very overwhelming if too much is consumed. So the low and slow approach is the way to start with oral dosing.

In contrast with the above, with some oils, such as CBD-rich hemp oils, you can start right off with rather large doses. The thing to keep in mind with legal CBD-rich hemp oils is this: CBD per milligram is expensive, currently, so cannabidiol is marketed in smaller sizes to keep the price down to where people will be more inclined to purchase it. If you purchase a 250mg bottle of CBD hemp oil, for instance, this could translate into only a few doses, depending upon the condition, and this translates to a costly substance for most at this level of dosing. Based on the current market price, as of this printing in summer 2015, CBD is around $50.00 to $80.00 for 250mgs. Things can certainly add up fast, depending upon your daily needs. You can get a bit better pricing in larger concentrations, but it is still a premium product in terms of cost. This will change when domestic hemp is approved for growing once again in the United States thereby reducing the need for imported hemp base.

The takeaway is this: Current sizing of hemp-based CBD products has more to do with attractive pricing than it does with actual therapeutic doses. The bottle might state, for instance, that it is a 30 or 60 day supply, but this is merely a labeling requirement: manufacturers must provide instructions so that a lay person has a reasonable expectation as to how to use the product.

Some children in Colorado suffering from epilepsy have started off at doses of cannabidiol around 4 to 6mg per pound of body weight, so a 250mg bottle would represent less than two doses at that rate for a 50-pound child. Epilepsy dosage rates of 300mg CBD a day or more have been reported.

I have seen studies for social anxiety where the single dose was 300 or 600mg. That is one dose of (typically synthetic) CBD for anxiety, a condition that most would rate as being less severe than a seizure. This is a substantial dose of CBD and the only side effect reported was slight drowsiness.

Furthermore, as another example, cannabis' effectiveness in cancer (according to some data) appears to be dose dependent, favoring higher doses, while still other studies point to a bell shaped response where a peak is reached, followed by diminishing returns at higher doses.

There is, by comparison, traumatic brain injury data in pigs that shows CBD activity NOT being dose dependent and, interestingly, similar neuroprotective results being found with either minute or large doses.

So this is all something to bear in mind. CBD oils, in particular, can be taken safely in large doses, and for some conditions, that might be desired. Still others might respond to as little as 5mg or 10mg doses a day. It is condition and individual dependent. There is no set rate or standardized dosing protocol.

In summary, cannabis oils with THC in them, to be safe, should be started slowly and increased gradually over time until the desired effect is achieved without unpleasant side effects, which, for most people, are nonexistent. Sleepiness, anxiety, paranoia, and dry eyes and mouth are probably the most frequent negative side effects for cannabis oils containing THC, but proper strain selection and sensible dosing can avoid much of this. CBD-rich hemp oils can be taken more liberally where the overall limiting factor in many cases in the actual cost of the oil.

Furthermore, I always advise when taking any new oil or tincture, it is wise to place a small drop on the skin or inner lip and wait for 30 minutes, observing for any swelling or itching that may indicate an allergy to something in the extract, as one can never tell what one might have an allergic reaction to. It is always better to be safe by testing first than sorry by taking a large initial dose and then having a reaction to it. I have personally had very mild allergic reactions to certain cannabis over the years, usually in the form of mild itching and swelling in the mouth, familiar symptoms to those that have had similar allergic reactions to foods, so it is just something to be aware of when trying new things. This is good practice in general, extending well beyond cannabis.


## Rick Simpson Dosing Protocol

The Rick Simpson regimen for cancer that many of you might have seen reference to online boils down to a very simple premise that goes along with what we have said before about low and slow. The idea with the Simpson protocol is to start off with low doses and slowly increase to the point that the user is taking essentially mega doses, completely saturating his/her system with the cannabinoids. If one were to take the ending doses when starting, it would be extremely uncomfortable, as people must build up tolerance to the effects of the cannabis in such large doses. So the idea is to slowly ramp up the cannabinoid levels in the body over the course of 4 to 8 weeks to allow the body to adjust to the effects while reaching a saturation point in the system with cannabinoid levels towards the end of dosing. This will help minimize any uncomfortable side effects from the substantially high ending doses of THC contained in the Rick Simpson style cannabis oils. That is really all there is to Rick Simpson protocol dosing in a nutshell. Rick Simpson style oils are marijuana-based, and users will experience a significant psychoactive effect at the doses required unless the dose is substantially buffered with the supplementation of a high CBD product, which can help temper some of the more intense effects by creating something closer to a 1:1 ratio of THC to CBD. This may, in fact, be an enhancement to the basic Simpson protocol that calls for *C. indica,* which, in some cases, can have very low levels of CBD in them. I do not personally make a distinction between *C. indicas* or *C. sativas* for making Simpson style cannabis oils for reasons of variance that we have covered in earlier chapters.

# Chapter 5

# The Best Ways to Consume Cannabis Medicinally

There are many ways in which cannabis can be consumed for medicinal benefit, and some options offer upsides that others lack. Let us take a look at some of the more common means of consuming cannabis and cannabis products.

## Smoking

Perhaps the most familiar and historically traditional method of consumption, smoking cannabis offers the benefits of immediate action with smoke taking around 8 seconds to hit the brain after inhalation. For conditions such as breakthrough pain, nausea and vomiting, and seizure and spasms, smoking cannabis offers the fastest relief possible—on par with injecting a substance directly into the body or vein.

Dry cannabis, oils, and concentrates can all be smoked, and the act of burning serves to decarboxylate the various substances making them more active in the body. The downside of this combustion process is that many things literally go up in smoke, and there is a fair amount of waste and byproduct; additionally, there are some toxins produced by combustion.

Smoking cannabis, however, seems to show none of the ill effects that tobacco smoke shows in studies. Cannabis smoke, due to its various active protective qualities, seems to mitigate much of the damage that comes from the act of smoking it. Long-term studies of heavy cannabis smokers, such as the one available here: http://www.scientificamerican.com/article/large-study-finds-no-link/, show no correlation in any increase in lung cancer or COPD risk, and in fact, some studies show prevalence rates lower than the non-tobacco smoking segment in the data.

## Vaporizing

Vaporizing cannabis is simply the act of using a device to heat the plant matter to a specific temperature whereby the active cannabinoids and terpenes are able to vaporize off the plant material without ever actually catching fire, producing a smokeless vapor that is low in tars and particulate matter. This process largely eliminates most of the toxins created by combustion and allows for precise temperature control for the vaporizing of certain cannabinoids and terpenes, which can sometimes be lost at the higher temperatures involved in smoking.

Clearly, vaporizing offers the speed of onset that smoking offers without the harms associated with smoke-related byproducts. The experience is different from smoking cannabis in effect on the body and mind, and consequently, some people prefer to smoke, while others prefer to vape, but many, in fact, do both. Both are effective means when immediate relief or effect is desired.

When purchasing a vaporizer, no expense should be spared and only high quality units constructed with heavy glass components with ceramic style heating elements should be chosen for maximum safety. Many cheaper units are constructed with various plastics and electronics that outgas into the same area that air is pulled through for inhalation, so just something to keep in mind when considering the $400.00 vaporizer versus the $40.00 pen unit. With vaporizers, in most cases, you get what you pay for with many of the more expensive models being well worth the investment. Many of the cheaper units are inefficient and possibly add toxins in the form of outgasses and metals released from the various heating elements used in cheaper units. One should look at hot points such as borosilicate glass, ceramic heating elements, and silicone tubing when shopping for vaporizers as well as precise temperature control.

With vaporizing, you are trading the potential toxins created with burning cannabis for the potential toxins created by the various metals used in the vaporizer heating elements as well as the plastic outgasses that can be created with many cheaper products. Vaporizers are not without their own set of inherent risks and downsides, though touted as a safer means of delivery than smoking. And if vaping pen style oils, such as the hemp-based CBD vape oils that can be found online, you are also vaporizing the various carrier agents and flavorings used in the production of commercial vape oils, which, in many cases, are the same as those used in e-cigs. All these are things to bear in mind when considering vaporizing as a method of ingestion.

## Dabbing Concentrates and Oils

Dabbing is the act of smoking/volatilizing very small doses of cannabis oil or concentrate on a specialized smoking device termed a dab rig. The vapor released is more of a vapor than a smoke due to the very high temperatures involved. A dab rig will, in its basic form, resemble a water bong with an added nail-like protrusion, which is composed of ceramic, titanium, glass, or quartz. This nail is heated to a red glow with a hand torch. Once the nail is heated, a small dab of concentrate is placed onto a metal or glass dabber and deposited onto the nail surface where it is immediately vaporized/volatilized and inhaled. Only very pure concentrate or oil should be smoked in this fashion. Dabbing gets its name from the saying that *a little dab will do ya*, alluding to the increased potency of the oils.

Dabbing has the benefit of being able to supply a *very* large dose in a very short time, which can be incredible for disorders such as the one I suffer from (Cyclical Vomiting Syndrome), when attacks come on in seconds. Nothing else I have found will completely derail the nausea like dabbing concentrate will. Pain, spasm, nausea —any breakthrough type issue—might benefit from the extreme potency and action of dabbing oils or concentrates.

In a nutshell, dabbing is a fantastic means of delivery when large doses and immediate action are needed.   While the visual of someone doing a dab with a hand torch might bring to mind hardcore drug use such as crack smoking, dabbing concentrate is a great way for those needing large doses of cannabis oils and should not be viewed as deviant or worrisome.

Again, if you decide to try dabbing, make sure the oil or concentrate you are using is designed to be dabbed and carefully prepared.  You do not want to dab oils or concentrates that are dirty with plant waxes and other residual matter/solvents.  If you are dabbing what are known as BHO or butane hash oil concentrates, be aware that butane is particularly effective at stripping the paraffin-like waxes from the *Cannabis* plant and that there is evidence that this can lead to a condition known as lipoid pneumonia when consumed   regularly.    This   condition   is   relatively   benign symptomatically, initially, until it becomes an issue, and then it really becomes an issue.  Pesticide residue is another large concern with concentrates and dabs, as the pesticides are concentrated to toxic levels in the extracts when present in the source *Cannabis* plants.

One potential downside of dabbing is a dramatic increase in tolerance due to the high levels of cannabinoids being ingested with each dab.    Those who dab chronically find themselves with ridiculous tolerance levels and many prior dabbers have since returned to smoking flowers only for recreational use.    For recreational users, dabbing might easily lead to abuse.  For medicinal users, there is no better method of administration for certain conditions, and it represents a valuable tool for delivery for those that need breakthrough relief.  Personally, I can smoke cannabis all day during one of my CVS flares, and it will not stop the vomiting. In fact, the act of smoking incurs even more vomiting for some people.  By contrast, I can take one dab and completely short circuit my nausea with oils from the proper strains.

Cancer patients attempting to achieve very high concentrations of cannabinoids in the body, may aslo possibly benefit from the very high doses achievable with this method of delivery.

We do not really know what the long-term effects of volatilizing cannabis oils are, as this is a relatively new technique, and if for no other reason than tolerance issues, I would caution against the overuse of dabbing as a delivery system and save it for times when it is really needed.

## Oral Dosing and Edibles

Cannabis oil can be eaten, and this is the preferred route of delivery for those seeking slow, extended release effects and steady blood serum levels. Cannabis oils are not water-soluble, so they often benefit from being mixed with a carrier oil, such as coconut or olive oil, to enhance their ability to be absorbed in the body.

Concentrated oil can be placed under the tongue for sublingual administration, as first pass metabolism through the liver is bypassed in this fashion, enhancing efficacy with less waste. One winds up losing a fair amount of beneficial substances due to the digestive process: as much as 80% can be lost. Though sublingual delivery is preferred if possible, holding oils in the mouth is sometimes impractical and hard to do once the saliva begins to flow.

These concentrated, sap-like oils can be mixed with a bit of olive or coconut oil to improve viscosity and absorbability, and then swallowed with other liquids or taken with food.

Anther popular way to imbibe thick oils is to pack them into gelcaps for easy dosing and elimination of off tastes from the cannabis oils.

Cannabis can be mixed with butter and filtered to create cannabutter—a very simple way to use cannabis in recipes in the kitchen. Cannabis can be cooked into just about anything that calls for oil or butter and does not require extreme heat because extreme heat might degrade the beneficial substances in the cannabis over time. Temperatures over 250 degrees Fahrenheit for more than 30 or so minutes are not recommended, unless a more sedative product is desired, as THC begins to convert to CBN at higher than 250 degrees Fahrenheit temperature. Through the use of both heat and time, this sedative property can be manipulated somewhat in the oven.


## Rectal Dosing/Suppositories

Rectal administration of cannabis oil has the benefit similar to sublingual delivery of bypassing the liver, skipping first pass metabolism, dramatically improving efficacy and the amount able to be absorbed from a given dose. You can find resources online (YouTube, etc.) that will show you how to make your own suppositories easily at home.

This method also has the advantage of putting the oil where it needs to go for folks with issues such as Crohn's, colitis, IBS, etc. Though not a popular route of administration, this is a legitimate means of delivery for cannabis oils and should not be discounted.


## Transdermal Dosing/Topical Salves

Transdermal dosing of cannabinoids also has the benefit of bypassing first pass metabolism and can be very effective for skin disorders such as psoriasis, lesions, cancers, and warts. Placing cannabis oil directly on a burn or wound or skin disorder could have dramatic results. Many companies produce topical salves, and there are even some that are starting to make transdermal patches available with various THC/CBD blends that are fantastic for slow, long-term release in the body.

The above methods represent the more common means of administering cannabis and cannabis oils. It is possible to use some or all of them in concert, and for some situations, a combination approach is often best. Smoking, vaping, and dabbing offer immediate onset and ease of dosing, whereas oral consumption offers slow release, more lasting effects, and steady levels of cannabinoids in the body. Sublingual, transdermal and rectal dosing offer the most efficient uptake and rapid onset when compared with oral dosing.

# Chapter 6

# CBD-Rich Hemp Oils

Recently, new arrivals on the cannabis scene are what are known as CBD-rich hemp oils. These are oils that are derived from industrial hemp plants, and as such, they are able to be fashioned into what are termed hemp finishing products, and can be imported and sold legally in the United States as well as many other countries that accept hemp imports. These hemp oils contain many of the same substances that marijuana strains contain with decent levels of CBD in them, especially when compared to marijuana oils, which have virtually zero CBD in them. It is important to note that CBD-rich hemp oils are almost entirely devoid of THC by virtue of being extracted from hemp strains.

Hemp oils offer one of the best methods of obtaining highly concentrated CBD at the moment and offer legal access to many of the other cannabinoids and terpenes found in marijuana strains that typically lack CBD content.

However, while these foreign industrial hemp plants have moderate levels of CBD in them, they are not high CBD cultivars raised for CBD production. Because of this, it takes more base material to provide a given concentration of cannabidiol. As more attention is placed on cannabidiol in the hemp industry, an increasing number of farms are starting to produce high CBD/low THC plants that qualify for hemp status under the law in order to fit the increasing need for high quality CBD hemp strains. This is happening especially in the U.S. right now with many states having implemented their own hemp growing programs that are focusing on producing high CBD hemp plants for cannabidiol extraction.

For instance, a foreign industrial hemp strain could come in at 2-3% CBD concentration. A domestic hemp/marijuana hybrid, however, might tip the scales at 20% CBD. It takes a lot less of the second plant to yield a given amount of extract and proportionally less man hours to raise a given number of plants for a given amount of extract.

The base material for these hemp oils can come from either the stalks of the plant or the entire plant. In general, one should seek out whole-plant extracts and full spectrum hemp oils that carry a full complement of cannabinoids and terpenes. Stalk-based extracts are expensive and require vast amounts of raw material, increasing the chance of concentrating any soil born contaminates into the final extract.

A few different solvents are commonly used in the industry for extractions, but super critical $CO_2$ is the cleanest method available. This method is also expensive but is a good indication the company producing the oil is not a fly-by-night operation. Ethanol extractions can also produce safe end products. I am happy to accept extracts of either type. The type of solvent used is one of the things I am looking for when evaluating a new oil with which I am unfamiliar.

Hemp oils are a legitimate source and, in fact, an excellent source, of high CBD oils at the moment, as marijuana oils are typically lacking any significant levels of CBD. Hemp-based CBD, as of this writing in mid-2015, is legal for purchase in the United States, as it is in over 40 other countries that allow for the sale of hemp products.

There has been a recent FDA ruling posted to a question and answer segment on the FDA official website wherein the FDA has stated that CBD is essentially reserved for a pharmaceutical company (GW Pharma) that has previously filed an investigational new drug (IND) application for its cannabis-based CBD pharmaceutical called Epidiolex. The hemp industry is expected to present evidence that, in fact, CBD has long been in the food supply and has been available in things such as hemp oils for decades, if not centuries.

At the time of the writing of this book, the FDA has not stated if it will move to shut down the otherwise legal CBD industry. One of the things the FDA looks for is if the substance in question is causing harm or loss of life. In the case of CBD, it is both non-intoxicating and nontoxic, and is a seemingly healthy substance to consume, while far more dangerous supplements remain on the market.

Whether this FDA ruling affects only those marketing pure CBD or extends into hemp oils remains to be seen. The current interpretation by many is that if the IND for GW Pharma were honored, it would only extend to pure CBD and not hemp oils.

Currently, CBD oils are available to purchase on Amazon, but they may contain no reference to cannabidiol (for whatever reason Amazon has determined to be the case). They must currently be labeled as simply hemp extracts to be sold. CBD had been available for purchase labeled as such via Amazon since at least 2013 without issue until they recently changed their policy on labeling requirements for merchants of CBD-rich hemp oils in the summer of 2015.

There are two bills pending this year: the Industrial Hemp Bill and the Charlotte's Web Therapeutic Hemp Act. These would remove both hemp and CBD from the controlled substances act once and for all in the United States. As such, 2015 is shaping up to be an interesting year to watch in regard to these issues.

There are dozens and dozens of companies marketing CBD-rich hemp oils today, and it pays to do a bit of research on these merchants. There are brands that are much better than others in terms of base materials being used, quality controls, and testing of their products. I would advise caution if shopping for hemp oils on sites such as Etsy, as many of the offerings are not, in fact, low THC legal offerings, and some are flat out just snake oil. Any website making bold health claims should be avoided, as this is a clear indicator that the seller is not in compliance with FDA regulations regarding supplements, and it makes you wonder what else the seller might not be compliant with.

It is a good idea to look for posted test data or to call and inquire about it personally. In fact, it is a good idea to call these companies as a part of your research. If they do not answer their phone or return calls in a timely manner, then that is another red flag. Companies offering legitimate products will be happy to talk to you about them.

And finally, beware of the vast amount of misinformation posted online with regard to hemp and hemp oils. There are people that will jump up and down, saying, *Hemp oil is not cannabis oil!* However, in fact, nothing can be further from the truth. There are those with a pro-THC legalization agenda that will accept nothing less than the whole-plant legalization of marijuana and will not consider the merits of anything short of that end goal.

Popular websites such as Project CBD and Ladybud have clear cut whole-plant agendas that skew their coverage of hemp oils considerably, and their stories get picked up by mainstream media, as their sites are considered so-called authority sites in light of the little or no competition in Google for the topic of cannabidiol. Most of the misinformation regarding hemp comes from those with little or no understanding about the actual genetics involved with various strains of *Cannabis*. These people would have you believe that there is nothing useful to be gained from high CBD hemp plants and that all patients with all illness need THC in their cannabis oil. This is simply not the case.

For those that do not need THC in their cannabis oils, high CBD hemp oils offer legal access to much of the *Cannabis* plant without the current legal specter that lurks over medical marijuana. You could take hemp-based CBD every day and not have to worry about failing an employment drug test. A parent can give hemp oils to their child and not have to worry about any unwanted psychoactive effects that might occur with marijuana oils. And even for those that *do* require THC, high CBD hemp oils offer the only way currently to easily obtain the CBD that most strains with THC are lacking so that they can also be used effectively to supplement marijuana oils, helping to reach that 1:1 golden ratio.


## Tips for Purchasing CBD-rich Hemp Oil Online

Try to procure *whole-plant* hemp oil versus stalk-based hemp extract.   Whole-plant hemp oil is more likely to have the full accompaniment of associated cannabinoid and terpenes.   Newer merchants are featuring whole-plant extracts, while older ones are still using stalk-based extracts, which are expensive and require vast amounts of raw material to yield any significant CBD concentrations.

Avoid merchants that feature prominent health claims, testimonials, or links to various cannabis studies.  All are against FDA regulations regarding herbal supplements, and any reputable company will be manufacturing and marketing their products according to industry guidelines.  There are many fly-by-night, just-pitched-their-tent companies hawking hemp-based CBD oils that do not take these regulations seriously.  Most studies that you will find linked on these companies' web pages actually reference studies done with either synthetic versions of the cannabinoids in question or the studies were done with full spectrum marijuana that also contained THC in addition to the CBD, so the bulk of these linked studies are misleading at best.

Assure that the company is adhering to both accepted Current Good Manufacturing Practice guidelines in their manufacturing facilities as well as adhering to the American Herbal Products Association standards.

Do not be afraid to try several brands.  As stated throughout this book, all cannabis and cannabis oil products are different, so if you do not see the results you are looking for from one oil, by all means, give another brand or two a try—remember: this is trial and error.

Reviews can be hard to find, as testimonials are not allowed to be posted for nutritional supplements for the most part, but there are websites such as Amazon.com that sell hemp-based CBD oils, that also feature product reviews, so this can be one source of information.  Keep in mind, though, that Amazon has been regularly removing and adding CBD oils from stock, so in many cases, these product reviews have been removed or not had a chance to build up over a year or so.

Start small.  Buy the smallest size offered—in many cases, 250mgs—and try that before investing in larger bottles.  Once you find a brand you like, you can typically get a bit of a price break by purchasing the larger sizes.  As previously stated, do not be afraid to try large doses (25, 50, 75, 100mg), depending upon what you are trying to treat.

Look for oils that have been extracted using super critical $CO2$.  This is both the cleanest method of extraction and the most expensive, indicating that the company is invested heavily in their manufacturing facilities or use a supplier for their base that has invested in this clean technology.  Almost all of the top companies offering hemp-based CBD oils are utilizing this technology now.

Be *very* careful on sites such as Etsy.  There are many, many smalltime producers of cannabis oils selling their goods on Etsy.  Be very aware that many of these offerings will not be legal for purchase if they were tested due to high THC levels.  Etsy is a popular marketplace but one I avoid when it comes to CBD oils.  There are many quality, legitimate vendors to be found on Etsy, but it is not worth filtering through the bad apples, in my estimation, unless you have a previous recommendation or tip.

Ignore most of the hemp hype you will encounter when looking for information regarding hemp-based CBD oils.  The vast majority of the commentary is without merit and without any basic understanding of the issues involved with producing cannabinoids from legal hemp plants.  Do not listen to the whole-plant rhetoric that you will need THC in your oils for them to be effective.  YOU will be the judge of this.  There are *many* folks who treat successfully with CBD oils and have little or no need for THC in their cannabis preparations.

    I personally run two informational blogs featuring recommendations to merchants whose products I have used firsthand myself and can recommend at cannabisoilforsale.net and cbdmarijuanaoil.com. There are many quality merchants selling hemp-based CBD oils online; one just needs to take a bit of time to shop around a bit to see what is out there.

# Chapter 7

# Producing Your Own Oil and Butter Safely

One of the best ways to assure the quality of the oils you are taking is to make them for yourself at home where you can closely keep tabs on the process and ensure a clean, safe end product. Please bear in mind that depending upon your location, making cannabis into a concentrated oil or edible product qualifies under separate concentrate laws that are often akin to crack cocaine laws and may carry absurdly stiff penalties in contrast to typical marijuana laws. I encourage anyone concerned with this to consult the state by state database at the National Organization for the Reform of Marijuana Laws (NORML) website for reference on specific state laws with regard to concentrates. This is the first and foremost safety consideration I can recommend. There have been people brought up on charges in various states just this last year for simply making marijuana brownies, so please exercise caution in this area.

Making your own oil might at first seem like a daunting task, but it can be rather simple and safe if done with the proper care. I strongly advise against the use of common solvents such as butane and naphtha—butane due to its highly explosive potential and naphtha due to its inherent toxicity.

In this chapter, we will examine some of the most common ways to safely produce cannabis oils at home and the methods that I feel are the most suited for folks new to cannabis oil extraction.


## A Word on Naphtha and Rick Simpson Oil

While researching cannabis oils, you might run across references to Rick Simpson oil (a popular method of making and consuming cannabis oil, often touted as an anti-cancer protocol). Simpson advocates the use of naphtha for extractions in his oil-making videos and reference materials. I would personally never recommend naphtha for use in making medicinal extracts, as folks with compromised immune systems cannot afford contamination from a residual solvent in their oils that can contain toxic substances such as benzene. Naphtha, a byproduct of the petroleum refining process, is, in fact, a soup of many chemicals—many of which are known carcinogens.

Simpson also advocates the use of *C. indica* strains exclusively, and this is questioned often. In reality, there is no real basis to use *C. indicas* over *C. sativas*, and in fact, as you learned in previous chapters, even finding pure versions of either species is a daunting task these days.

As discussed in previous chapters, ALL *Cannabis* plants are capable of producing the same substances under the right conditions. I would concern myself with procuring high quality marijuana, first and foremost, of any heritage, be it *C. indica* or *C. sativa* or hybrid. If you can find strains that are reasonably high in CBD as well, this would be a bonus, but simply seeking *C. indica* strains is not enough to accomplish this.

## A Brief Word on Decarboxylation

In general, when extracting oils from cannabis, one should consider the process of decarboxylation. Decarboxylation refers simply, in layman's terms, to the activation of the cannabinoids contained within the cannabis oil into forms that are readily available to our receptors through processes of heating, drying, or curing. When cannabis is decarboxylated, it transforms key cannabinoids such as THCa and CBDa in fresh cannabis into their decarboxylated versions of THC and CBD. Referring back to the chapter on cannabinoids, recall there are separate effects attributed to the different versions of these cannabinoids.

The basic premise behind decarboxylation is that *any* heating of cannabis in the range of 200 to 250 degrees Fahrenheit for 20 to 30 minutes (be it via cooking or during the removal of solvents during the oil making process) will accomplish the end result of decarboxylating the cannabis fully and activation of the cannabinoids.

Cannabis should ideally be cured (carefully dried) for a minimum of 8 to 12 weeks after being cut from the plant. Fresh cannabis should be stored in a container that promotes evaporation, such as a wooden cigar box or a paper bag for the duration of the curing process (after initially being line dried to the point of the stems snapping when attempting to break one). Freshly harvested cannabis should not be stored in plastic bags or containers that promote sweating or moisture retention, nor should cannabis be stored in the freezer where moisture cannot leave the flowers.

Once cannabis has been thoroughly cured, it can then be placed into more airtight containers for long-term storage. It is also perfectly fine to slow cure cannabis in canning jars, opening the lid every now and again to let the air exchange a bit. Again, the cannabis should be dry enough for the stems to snap before placing it in the canning jar for long-term curing/storage. There are many more ways to cure cannabis, but the paper bag and canning jar methods are traditional methods that yield good results.

Cannabis that has been cured properly for many months in this fashion will have no need for further decarboxylation, as this happens naturally as part of this slow curing process. For many reasons though, much marijuana that is sold has not been cured for the proper amount of time, which necessitates further decarboxylation for maximum potency.

The only reason one would *not* want to decarboxylate their cannabis at some point in the extraction process would be if they were seeking more of the acid versions of the cannabinoids such as THCa and CBDa or seeking to produce an oil that is less psychoactive in the end. The preservation of terpenes with low boiling points would be another reason not to decarboxylate a cannabis oil.

One can control the amount of psychoactivity in the oils they produce to some extent by utilizing differing degrees of decarboxylation during the extraction process. If the goal is to produce a less psychoactive oil, simply decarb for a shorter amount of time, thus converting less THCa into THC. Conversely, if the goal were to produce a more sedative oil, the process of heating should be carried on longer than 30 minutes, which will result in THC being further converted into CBN, producing a more sedative, less psychoactive oil. Contrary to popular belief, THC does not degrade into CBD when heated: only CBN can be created this way.

If you wish to achieve maximum potency from the cannabis and also wish to use quick methods of making the oil, it is a good idea to go ahead and decarb the marijuana first. If you know for a fact that the cannabis has had a good long and proper cure, then decarbing will not be necessary. Please note, though, that due to greed, most street marijuana is sold damp to increase profits where water equals weight. Unless you live in a legal state with retail access to well-cured product, most marijuana purchased on the black market will need to be decarbed, especially if you want to use right away, as it will not have been cured adequately to begin with.

Freshly harvested cannabis can be decarboxylated very simply in an oven. If the cannabis is *very* wet or fresh, allow it to room cure in an open container for a week to 10 days, if possible, until it reaches a state of being able to snap the stems cleanly. At this point, it will then be ready for the oven and decarboxylation.

I strongly advise again quick drying methods for very fresh cannabis and recommend a food dehydrator be used if rapid drying of freshly harvested cannabis must be accomplished. A food dehydrator will be able to dry fresh cannabis in 4 to 6 hours time.

Patience is a virtue with regard to curing cannabis properly. Rushing the curing process will result in bitter and off tastes in both edible or smoked cannabis and might dramatically impact the potency of the final product.

## To Decarboxylate Cannabis in the Oven

Using a glass pie plate or similar container (avoid metal cookie sheets that might scorch), crumble the herb into a thin layer and place into a preheated oven at 220 degrees Fahrenheit for 25 to 30 minutes. After this, the herb will be decarboxylated and ready for use in the preparation of oils.

If cannabis oils or extracts are to be used in cooking and, therefore, will be exposed to heat in the 225 to 350 degree Fahrenheit range, this is usually enough to decarboxylate the material thoroughly. However, if cannabis oils are done as cold extractions, then prior decarboxylation of the herb is often desired to achieve maximum potency and activity in the end oil.

Generally, when making cannabis oils, the process of boiling off the solvent during extraction or using the oil for cooking will be more than enough to decarboxylate the extraction. However, it is important to be aware of the decarboxylating process and how it can be manipulated to produce oils that contain different ranges of cannabinoids, or levels of psychoactivity, depending upon what the ultimate goal of the patient is.

## A Brief Word on Kief

Kief, hash, or hashish, refers to the sifted and collected resin glands from the *Cannabis* plant. In the same way that a solvent can be used to remove the resin glands from the leaf material, mechanical means can also be used to dislodge the glands, which are then filtered and collected to form a powder that is known as kief. Think of kief as essentially powdered cannabis oil.

Kief is sometimes preferred for making oils and concentrates, as it has already had the vast majority of plant material removed, leaving only the sifted resin glands behind for concentration. This usually makes for more timely and efficient extractions.

Kief is created easily, though it requires a fair amount of cannabis to produce a small amount of kief. The easiest way to make kief is to just use a fine screen (a grease screen usually used to protect from splatters over a frying pan works fantastically for this) and very dry herb. Break the cannabis up into small pieces (but not too fine) and simply place the cannabis on the screen over a clean surface or large piece of paper, and thump it, repeatedly, dislodging the glands that will then fall through the screen onto the collection surface. After this, the glands can then be scraped up into a pile with a credit card or similar item. This thumping process is continued until little kief falls from the remaining cannabis in the screen. The cannabis that has been thoroughly shaken can then be used for further cooking or extraction, but will have lost most of what makes it potent to the hash-making process and may simply be discarded as well.

Another simple way to make kief is to take very dry herb, break it up (not to the point of powder but into small pieces) and place into a plastic food container in the freezer to freeze overnight. If you can find dry ice, this makes things even easier. Place a few tiny chunks of dry ice in the container the next day with the frozen cannabis and shake it vigorously for 4 or 5 minutes. If you do not have dry ice, just shake the frozen cannabis in the container. When finished shaking, sift the herb through a fine mesh screen such as a silkscreen, nut milk bag, or nylon paint strainer. A screen of around 100 to 200 microns is fine for this; larger sizes up to 600 microns work well but will allow for more vegetative material to collect. (I like to use a mesh grease screen to do an initial sifting and then run that material through the fine screen for a final sifting.)

The freezing process causes the resin glands to become brittle, allowing them to easily slough off of the plant surfaces. (Again, if you cannot get dry ice, just simply freeze the herb in the plastic container and then shake and filter the result several times until you stop getting kief.) A benefit of the plastic container is that it will create a small static charge when shaking the frozen cannabis, which will attract the resin glands onto the surfaces of the container where you can use your finger to easily gather them up. Pour the cannabis from the container onto the screen for sifting, clean off the surfaces of the container with your finger, and return the cannabis to the container and refreeze for at least an hour or so. Repeat the entire process until you stop getting decent returns of kief, at which point the remaining leaf/bud material may be discarded or used for further cooking or extraction, but most of the resin glands will have been removed at this point, diminishing the quality of the remaining plant material.

A paper bag can be used with the dry ice method instead of a plastic container or what are known as Bubble Bags (designed for hash making) can be purchased online and used for shaking/sifting as well.

Another method of collecting kief is what is known as ice water hash. This method works really well with leaf trim and waste products from the harvest of fresh cannabis. The method is as follows: Place previously frozen dried leaf material in a large container or bucket filled with water and much ice. You want a nice layer of ice, but you do not want to fill the entire container with ice, just enough to provide a nice top layer a couple inches deep on top of the water. Using a hand blender, agitate this mixture for anywhere from 15 minutes to an hour. Allow this to settle for 5 minutes and then remove the floating ice and leaf from the surface of the water with your hand to discard. Next, pour and filter this liquid through a 100 to 200 micron-sized screen into a large glass measuring cup or glass bowl. A clear plastic container will work fine for this as well. I like to use a clear container with see through sides for this step so that I can see the layer of kief on the bottom when viewing from the side of the container. A container that gets progressively smaller toward the bottom, such as a large glass measuring cup, will also help to gather the kief into a nice layer as it settles. A mesh grease screen or nylon paint strainer works very well as a screen for this step. The green leafy material trapped on top of the screen or strainer can be discarded.

Allow this drained liquid to settle for 10 minutes and a layer of kief will form at the bottom of the container. Before it forms at the bottom, it will look like sandy snow falling from suspension in the water. Using a turkey baster, syringe, or other suitable device, remove or siphon off the water layer from on top of the kief layer on the bottom of the container, being careful not to disturb the settled kief on the bottom. You can also pour the liquid through a standard coffee filter and collect the kief that way from on top of the filter, scraping it up gently with a credit card after the liquid has drained away. Form a ball or pile of this kief and allow this to further air dry for a day or two, allowing the rest of the water to evaporate off. A paper towel rolled into a tight tube and left to rest on the kief is helpful for wicking up the remaining water. It is ready for use when dry and powdery.

Bubble Bags that are especially designed for this purpose are also readily available online and are designed to fit around standard bucket sizes. Bubble bags offer a series of progressively smaller filter bags to allow for the very fine separation of kief. If using a Bubble Bag system for making ice water hash, I recommend a quick look at YouTube for the many videos that are posted on the subject to get an idea of how others use them for hash separation.

Kief collected in these manners can then be used for further purification into oil without the worry of substantial amounts of chlorophyll coming off of the plant matter, which can lead to gastric distress in those who are sensitive to chlorophyll. The other benefit of this approach of turning cannabis into kief first is that much less solvent is needed to cover kief as opposed to the amount of cannabis the kief was shaken off of. There are definite benefits to working with kief over whole cannabis in the preparation of oils. The major downside is that it takes a fair amount of cannabis to create a small amount of kief—approximately 7- 10 grams of dry cannabis to yield one gram of kief for average quality marijuana.

## Cannabutter

One of the oldest traditional methods of cannabis oil preparation is making a simple cannabis butter. This method is both safe and easy to incorporate into meals. It is very simple to make with just butter and marijuana being all that is needed, and while there are quite a few variations on this basic process, here is the method that I prefer:

First off, clarify the butter into what is commonly known as ghee. This will remove many of the unsavory solids and undesirables from the butter, leaving a nice, clear, end product.

Clarification process of butter to ghee: Use unsalted butter. Heat the butter on medium-high heat until it comes to a boil and then back the heat off to medium, and let it cook. The butter will foam up and then appear to stop foaming. Wait for it to foam up again. When the butter foams up again for the second time, it is done cooking. This will take approx 6 to 8 minutes, depending upon the stove.

Allow the butter to cool for a few minutes and then strain it through cheesecloth. Alternately, pour the melted butter into a glass measuring cup or container and refrigerate it until solidified. At this point, the butter will have formed distinct layers, and you can remove the clarified butter from off of the top of the solids, which will have precipitated out to the bottom of the container. Either way, the clarified butter is now ready to be combined with the cannabis for the next step.

For the next stage, either prepare a sachet or just add the cannabis directly to the butter in the cooking vessel. A double boiler setup or crock-pot works well for the cooking. I prefer to add the cannabis directly to the butter in order to maximize surface contact, but alternatively, you can also take several layers of cheesecloth and wrap the cannabis up into a tidy sachet tied with some cooking string, etc. The prepared cannabis should be crumbly dry, but not powdery and either placed into the sachet or directly into the butter.

The cannabis can be previously decarbed as described earlier or a longer cooking time can be used to accomplish this same process—either way is fine. If further baking is to be done with the cannabutter after preparation, reduce the cooking time in this step somewhat to prevent too much THC loss to conversion by the time the second round of heating is done with the baking of the final cookies or whatever you might be using the cannabutter for.

Use a ratio of 1/4 ounce cannabis to one stick of butter or one 1/2 cup clarified ghee. Place the butter/ghee and cannabis/sachet into a crock-pot or double boiler setup on the stovetop and let it cook for several hours at low heat. If it is in the crock-pot, let it go on low for 12 to 24 hours.

Once time is up, remove the sachet, if one was used, and squeeze the remaining butter out from it. If a sachet was not used and the cannabis is mixed with the butter, strain said mixture through several layers of cheesecloth to remove the solid plant matter. Pour this strained butter into a final glass bowl or storage container and place in the fridge to cool. This cannabutter is now ready to eat as is. It can be slowly dissolved in the mouth or used in place of butter in any traditional recipe.

There are many variations on this basic method. I encourage those interested in making cannabutter to utilize YouTube to check out a few different videos, which will allow you to find a method that works best for your kitchen, supplies, time, etc. If you are making small batches, add a cup of water or so also to the butter at the start, to keep things from drying out a bit. This water is later removed after cooling, where it will stratify into a separate layer. This method also helps remove some of the more bitter water-soluble components of the cannabis, making the end product a bit more palatable. Some use the water, some skip it; it is up to your preference.

## Infused Cooking Oils

Many cooking oils make excellent carriers for fat-soluble

cannabinoids, and as such, they also make great solvents for extracting the resins from the plant matter efficiently. Oils such as coconut and olive are preferred due to their saturated fat content, but any vegetable or nut oil can be used, e.g., hemp seed oil, almond oil, apricot oil, etc.

Preparation of these oils is very much like preparing cannabutter. The cannabis can be decarboxylated prior to adding it to the oil if one wishes for a faster cook time or just combine the oil with the cannabis, letting it cook at low-medium temperature for 4 to 6 hours, minimum.

An easy way to make infused oils is to use a standard canning jar. Fill the jar around half full with the prepared dry cannabis and then add the oil of choice to cover the herb by 1 1/2 to 2 times the level of the cannabis. Place this jar into a water bath in a small saucepan on the stove with a lid loosely screwed on top, leaving it loose enough to vent any vapor that wants to escape during the cooking process. Place a spare canning lid or something similar on the bottom of the saucepan to keep the canning jar containing the cannabis/oil mixture from touching the bottom of the saucepan, which could potentially cause the jar to crack when heating.

Let this simmer on low heat, just under a boil for as long as is practical, anywhere from 6 to 24 hours. If you need to go to sleep or leave the house, you may just let the jar sit on the cold stove until you can resume heating again later. You cannot mess this stage up: simply make sure that you try to achieve at least 6 hours of total heating time at a minimum. Less time is required if the cannabis was previously decarboxylated. Add pre-warmed water to the saucepan as necessary as it evaporates during the day, being careful not to pour much cooler water onto the canning jar when adding it, potentially cracking the jar.

Strain this oil after cooking and cooling through several layers of cheesecloth, or I like to use nylon paint strainers that are readily found in most hardware paint sections.

Store the oil in a dark cupboard and take it as needed. It can be used as a topical, taken by the spoonful, or added to recipes in place of cooking oil. If using coconut oil as a base, the oil might need to be defrosted by warming the container of oil in a warm water bath, to return the oil to a liquid state for easy administration or use in recipes, as coconut oil tends to solidify under 75 degrees Fahrenheit.

## Tinctures: Green Dragon

Alcohol-based tinctures are efficient means of delivery, and there is a bit of a synergistic effect that occurs when alcohol is used as a carrier in terms of absorbability. Homemade tinctures can be very strong and efficacious, and one of the old standbys is something known as Green Dragon tincture.

Green Dragon is made with 190 or 151 proof alcohol, usually rum or Everclear. A proof of 190 will allow for more alcohol to be evaporated off, making a stronger tincture, where 151 will have more alcohol left in it in the end. Kief, or powdered hash is preferred, especially with 151, but dry cannabis buds can be used, as well.

## Method for Green Dragon from Dry Cannabis

Decarb 1/4 ounce cannabis, per previous instructions in the section on decarboxylation. Place it into a small canning jar and freeze overnight; place the bottle of alcohol in the freezer, as well. The next day, add 3 fluid ounces of the frozen alcohol to the herb, shake for a good 5 minutes gently, and then return the jar to the freezer for a couple more hours. After this, shake for a few more minutes and then pour the contents through a wire mesh filter or cheesecloth— something that will catch the bulk of the large pieces but still drain the liquid quickly into a glass bowl or suitable container. Cheesecloth is nice in that you can pick it up and wrap the herb to squeeze out the remaining liquid easier. A nylon paint filter also works well for this, readily available in the paint sections of most hardware stores.

Squeeze out excess alcohol through the mesh or cheesecloth and either return this plant material to the freezer for a second wash or discard it at this point. If you are doing a second wash, simply repeat the first step over for the additional wash using half the amount of alcohol. This will ensure a more complete extraction of the cannabis and pick up what was not washed out of the first run.

Take this filtered liquid and pour it through a coffee filter, allowing it to slowly drain into a suitable glass jar or container. A metal funnel can be used to hold the filter or the filter can be tied to the top of whatever container being used to drain the extract into. To eliminate filter loss, cut the filter down to the needed size, and dip it in a small shot glass of alcohol, wringing it out prior to use or use a cooking brush to brush some alcohol onto the filter. This will keep the extract liquid from absorbing into the dry coffee filter as much as possible, which helps keep the extracted oil from being lost to the filter while draining.

Next, reduce the amount of alcohol a bit. With 151, you cannot reduce it very much due to the water content, but with 190 proof, you can reduce it by half. Do this by simply setting the open jar into a nice warm sunny spot outside and just let it slowly evaporate until it reduces. Cover the opening with a piece of cheesecloth or something similar to keep any dust out while it is evaporating.

Alternatively, use a water bath in a saucepan. Place the jar with the Green Dragon mixture into a small saucepan on top of the stove. Be sure to keep the jar off of the bottom of the saucepan with an extra canning jar lid or something similar. Fill the saucepan with water to the approximate level of the green dragon liquid in the jar.

This is best done outside with adequate ventilation on a portable electric burner, but if you are doing this on a stove top, make sure it is an electric range and that there are no ignition sources or open flames, have the doors and windows open, a fan running, and just use common sense. Again, it is best to go outside.

Slowly bring the water bath up to temp in the saucepan. The alcohol will start boiling off at around 170 degrees Fahrenheit and should be left to boil until the desired level is reached—in this case, a 50% reduction. Using an oven mitt or glove, carefully remove the jar of Green Dragon from the water bath.

The tincture is now ready for use. Be careful, this can be *very* strong: start off with several *drops* and wait a couple hours. Slowly increase until you find your dosage. It should be mixed with juice or water, as it will burn by itself. I recommend putting a small drop on your lip and waiting 30 minutes to check for swelling, itching, burning, etc., in case any odd allergies, etc., appear. Keep in mind, the strong alcohol will burn by itself, so do not mistake that for an allergic reaction. You can always test a drop of alcohol first (before testing the tincture) to gauge what the burn is like from just the alcohol alone.

## Method for Green Dragon from Kief

Decarb the kief as described earlier and make sure it is broken up well. Place the kief into small canning jar and add 1/2 fluid ounce alcohol to 1 gram of kief ratio. If you do not have a scale, simply add enough alcohol to cover the kief by roughly an inch or two. Shake the jar well and allow it to set for an hour. Next, filter the mixture through a small coffee filter cut to size and pre-wet with alcohol (the same as described above). After this, the tincture is ready for use. Remember to go slow and start with low doses.

You can reduce the alcohol as above, if desired. Essentially, reducing the alcohol at the end just increases concentration per drop of tincture. It is totally up to you as to how much you want to let naturally evaporate or boil off. Also, reducing the alcohol presents more cannabis with less alcohol in the equation, but bear in mind that a half dozen drops of alcohol will not provide much of an effect in terms of an unwanted side effect from the alcohol.

## Hash Oil/Cannabis Oil

There are many ways to make pure cannabis oils: all involving the use of a solvent of one type or another and of varying degrees of safety with regard to these particular types of solvents. I would strongly urge against the home use of solvents such as butane, naphtha, or hexane due to either issues with toxicity or explosivity, especially in light of the availability of safer alternatives for amateur extractions.

Alcohol extractions are typically much safer for amateurs, and while still requiring fresh air, ventilation, and a good dose of common sense, they are not as volatile as working with solvents such as butane.

You will want to have a decent quality digital laser type thermometer on hand for precise temperature measurement during the reduction process involved with making these types of cannabis oils. These may be purchased cheaply and easily on Amazon.com. I would personally not attempt to carry out this type of extraction without one.

When it comes to alcohol, there are two choices: 190 proof Everclear/ethanol, equivalent, or 99% pure isopropyl alcohol. Lesser proof alcohol/ethanol or isopropyl cannot be used due to the amount of water found in lower proof drinking alcohols and possible denaturing agents used in lower percent isopropyl. Everclear has the advantage of being a food grade solvent that, while still being considered toxic, is consumed routinely by many for recreational purposes. Isopropyl is toxic in significant doses, as are the vapors, but is safe for oil extraction as long as proper care is taken to purge all residual solvent from the oil at the end of the process. Make certain that the isopropyl alcohol has not been denatured, as the denaturing agents added to make the products undrinkable are toxic.

The process for making cannabis oil with either type of alcohol is very similar.

In making oil, either dry cannabis or kief can be used. The cannabis should be dry enough to break up into small fragments but not dry enough to crumble into dust. If necessary, bake the herb on a thin layer in the oven briefly to reach the desired dryness. I prefer to use a glass container for 10 or 15 minutes at 200 degrees Fahrenheit. Afterward, place the still warm cannabis into an appropriate-sized canning jar/s (jars should be filled to about 50% level with cannabis to allow room to add the alcohol later) and place the jar/s as well as the bottle of alcohol in the freezer for at least 24 hours. This will help to lock up any remaining water present in the cannabis.

The next process will vary, depending upon whether isopropyl or Everclear is used in terms of how long to soak the herb in the alcohol. These methods are what are known as quick wash extractions, and the time is carefully monitored to prevent the stripping off of less desirable elements such as plant waxes and chlorophyll.

If using Everclear, do a 3-minute wash. Add the chilled alcohol to the canning jar with the frozen cannabis to a level a few inches above the cannabis and shake well or stir with a butter knife to make sure all surfaces are wet. Return the jar to the freezer and wait for 3 minutes. After that, remove the jar from the freezer and give the jar one last shake or stir and pour the contents through a wire mesh strainer—one that is small enough to trap most of the large pieces of plant matter but large enough to allow the alcohol to drain off quickly into an appropriate glass vessel or stainless steel measuring cup.

Squeeze any remaining liquid from the material through the strainer with a spoon or something similar to compress the mass. This cannabis is then either discarded or returned to the freezer for refreezing where you can repeat the same process again for a second or third wash. The first wash will remove about 75% of the cannabinoids with the second and third washes producing less and less for the added effort and solvent.

If using isopropyl alcohol, the process is the same but the wash time is reduced to a mere 20 seconds, as Isopropyl is 99% alcohol and acts very rapidly to dissolve the plant resins. Longer soak times will result in more contaminants being picked up such as waxes and chlorophyll that will turn the oil from amber to green or black.

Again, the cannabis can be refrozen and washed the same way 2 or 3 times for maximum extraction. More washes will pull more unwanted plant contaminates as well, so bear that in mind.

If using kief instead of herb in the above scenarios, slightly longer soak times can be used in both cases, as much of the plant material will have already been removed, minimizing the chances of picking up undesirable plant extracts. That will be the only difference in the process when using kief—longer soak times. For instance, kief can sit for 2 or 3 minutes in isopropyl versus the 20 seconds for dry herb. A soak time of 3 to 5 minutes will also be adequate with 190 proof when using kief.

From here, we take our roughly filtered alcohol mixture and prepare it for the final filtration. This mixture will be filtered through a standard unbleached coffee filter into a suitable stainless steel container. I recommend the stainless container be large enough to accommodate twice the amount of liquid you will be filtering into the cup, e.g., for 1/2 cup of liquid, use a minimum size of a 1 cup container. Cone shaped coffee filters and a stainless steel funnel can be used as well for this purpose. Cut off the excess filter to prevent liquid from absorbing into the extra filter material and place into the funnel to hold in place. The filter may be prewet with a bit of 190 or isopropyl to cut down on filter absorption loss. Pour the extract through this filter and allow to slowly drain into the stainless cup.

Alternatively, place the coffee filter directly over the mouth of the cup the extract is poured into and use some hemp string or something similar to secure it to the top of the cup. Make a depression in the filter before tying the string to form a small bowl and pour the liquid in over a few separate pours, waiting for the fluid level to drain between each one, being careful not to drip and spill. If you are a bit sloppy by nature, just get yourself a funnel to hold the filter! Also make sure the metal cup the mixture is draining into is deep enough so that the filter can form a shallow bowl without touching the liquid below as it fills (if you are tying the filter directly on to the mouth of the stainless container).

Either way, pour the liquid carefully through the coffee filter, allowing it to slowly drain. An extra trick is to use a nylon paint strainer or nut milk bag to place over the coffee filter while you pour the alcohol through, allowing you to wrap up the larger plant material into a tight bundle when you are done draining it in order to squeeze out all the remaining liquid efficiently onto the coffee filter below. This also helps keep all the bigger particles from clogging up the coffee filter, slowing down the draining process.

Once the extract is filtered, you are now ready to reduce all of the alcohol out of it.

You will want to carry out this process using a double boiler setup or, alternatively, a rice cooker can be used. I will explore the double boiler method. I would advise that this step be carried out outdoors or in a kitchen with superior stove top ventilation to the exterior of the house (not the recirculating filter style fans). If inside, all doors and windows should be opened and extra care taken to deal with any vapors, which, in the case of isopropyl, are toxic to breathe. You must use your common sense here. If you can smell fumes, there is likely a flash hazard. Have an extinguisher on hand and have a way to cover the pan in the event of a grease fire, as you will be using cooking oil for the bath in the double boiler because of needing to raise the temperature of the bath beyond the boiling point of water.

A simple cheap portable electric burner unit that can be purchased for 15 or 20 dollars works well for outdoor use. When using this style of cheap burner, you will simply be turning it on for a few mins, and then turning it back off, as most of these units have very poor temperature control. You will repeat the on/off process every 5 mins or so throughout in order to maintain your heat where you want it. You will be using a 250 degree Fahrenheit oil bath, so you will be dealing with hot oil and alcohol: care MUST be taken! Make sure the container used to boil the extract off with cannot tip over in the saucepan of cooking oil it will be placed into!

I prefer a small narrow saucepan for this (the single burner size).

Place an extra canning lid or something similar into the bottom of the saucepan; this will keep the cup with the extract from coming into contact with the saucepan. This is the basic double boiler setup. Anything that can be immersed in hot oil to hold the cup an half inch or inch or so off of the bottom of the saucepan is fine to use here— washers, jar lids, etc. Just make sure whatever is used provides a solid base for the stainless cup with the extract to sit on.

Fill the saucepan with cooking oil to about the same level the extract level will be be in the stainless cup (once it is sitting in the saucepan). For instance, if there are 2 inches of extract in the stainless cup and a half inch lid placed under it to keep it raised off the bottom of the saucepan, add about 2 ½ inches of cooking oil to the saucepan, overall. This will help to keep the cup from floating and becoming a little boat, if you will, as the alcohol evaporates, which could lead the cup to capsize, ruining the oil! Do not let this happen to you, as it can happen in a snap, wasting all of your time and effort as well as your precious oil.

Make sure the stainless cup is secure on top of whatever it raised on top of and not tippy in the least when sitting in the cooking oil. The heavier the metal cup, the better, as lighter ones might float as the alcohol level is reduced inside it. You will get a feel for this; it can be a bit tricky your first time through. If you have something a bit heavy that can straddle the top of the container to help weigh it down a bit, such as a small wrench or tool, that can also be helpful.

Key points: Get as heavy a stainless cup as possible, do not fill the saucepan with oil above the level of extract in the stainless cup, and make sure the stainless cup is raised off of the bottom of the saucepan and stable in the oil bath.

Slowly raise the temperature of the cooking oil to 220-ish degrees Fahrenheit. The alcohol will start to boil as it reaches around 170 to 180 degrees Fahrenheit. All of the alchohol must be evaporated before the oil will come up in temperature to the 220 range to boil off the remaining water in the oil, so dont be alarmed if the oil will not rise over 170 initially, while the cooking oil bath is

220 degrees.    Avoid breathing the vapors as the alcohol boils off. Using a laser thermometer is a good way to keep an eye on the temperature of both the cooking oil bath and the alcohol mixture during this process.  Keep the cooking oil bath no more than around 220-225 degrees Fahrenheit.

Once the alcohol is reduced, the remaining water will then almost instantly boil off and the rolling boil will stop and you will be left with a brownish amber concentrate that is producing many pea sized small bubbles. At this point, you can finish the process on the stove indoors if you would like, being very careful if transferring and moving back inside not to trip or spill the container!  You will be cooking the oil for an additional 15 to 30 minutes, so I tend to move back inside to the stove for this step.  This step WILL stink up the house like marijuana as many terpenes will evaporate during this stage, so if smell is an issue, carry on outdoors.

While the very last bits of alcohol cook off, keep a close eye on the temperature of the reduced oil in the stainless cup, which should not exceed 250 degrees Fahrenheit.   Ideally, strive for a uniform layer of oil across the bottom of the cup 1/8 inch or so in depth.  If it is a small batch, tilting the container slightly with a metal washer or something to shim one side of the cup slightly from below, will allow you to create a small pool on one side of the cup 1/8 inch in depth or so.   This will help ensure the last traces of alcohol are removed.  Do not let the oil become thin and dry on the surface of the cup, or the alcohol will become difficult to liberate from it and as well, it should not be much more than an 1/8 inch or so in depth.

Raise the heat a bit to med-low and allow the cannabis oil in the stainless cup to come up to 250 degrees Fahrenheit in temperature and simmer it until all bubbling has stopped—usually about 15 minutes or so. At first, there will be larger bubbles that then start to turn into very small pinhead bubbles.  Once the oil is still and there is nothing but the very occasional tiny pinhead bubble forming in the oil, it is ready to be removed for cooling.  Do not allow the cannabis oil in the stainless cup to go over 250 degrees Fahrenheit during this stage or THC content will rapidly diminish. Remove the cup carefully from the oil bath and set it aside to cool. The cannabis oil is ready for use after cooling.

This method will produce some of the purest cannabis oil possible. As long as care is taken to evaporate all traces of alcohol, it is suitable for dabbing and smoking as well as being taken orally. The oil will be the consistency of very thick honey or pinesap, so it can be packed into gelcaps for ease of swallowing or thinned back down again with a cooking oil such as olive or coconut to make the oil easier for the body to digest and easier to handle. Time release gelcaps that release further down in the GI tract make excellent choices for delivery, eliminating some of the loss from stomach acids.

The more amber the color of the oil, the less contaminated it is with other plant substances.

While there are many other methods of producing cannabis extracts, the ones above are the ones I feel are the easiest for most amateurs to do at home safely. I advise spending some additional time on YouTube to see variations on these techniques from others before attempting for the first time, as it is always helpful to watch someone do it first. You can also find small variations in technique that fit your particular situation or available tools more than others. All methods will employ the same basic process, but you will find folks have little personal tricks for some of the steps, such as filtering, etc., so watching some videos can be really helpful for the uninitiated.

Always exercise proper common sense and basic safety when working with things such as flammable alcohol vapors, and always take the time to make sure that you are properly purging all traces of the alcohol from the finished cannabis oil by using proper heat for the proper amount of time, while carefully watching and monitoring the formation of bubbles in the oil. All but the tiniest pinhead bubbles should be gone in the final heated cannabis oil, indicating that all of the alcohol has been boiled off, and there should be no residual odor of alcohol left.

If any of these steps or methods make you squirm too much or you feel nervous about executing them, please do not attempt them! You *can* burn yourself or your house *severely* if proper safety precautions are not observed during this process, and you can expose yourself to toxins in your oil if you do not properly purge the alcohol off in the last step. If you take your time, consult some video references, and practice safety, making your own cannabis oil is quite simple.

For more information on every way possible to extract cannabis oils and detailed methodology for extractions, I recommend the excellent pages over at the Skunk Pharm Research website.

## Extra: Pro Tips for Cleanup

The residue from the alcohol mixes are a bit like superglue and will form a varnish on all surfaces it comes into contact with! The only way to get it off of utensils is to either use more alcohol or use cooking oil. I simply wash the vessels and utensils with a sponge dipped in some kind of cooking oil first (this will dissolve the cannabis residues). Then just use simple dish soap to remove this oil from the dishes. I do the same thing to clean my hands: just use a bit of cooking oil on dry skin and then dish soap to remove the oil. The residual oil left on the surfaces of the stainless steel cup used for reducing the cannabis oil is retrieved by rubbing a couple of teaspoons of cooking oil onto the cup and collecting the result, which can then be taken orally or mixed with food. I do this when I have used up the last of my oil, as I tend to store my oil in the reduction cup to prevent transfer losses when moving it to another container.

# Chapter 8

# Conclusion

In conclusion, it is my hope that this book has helped to demystify the *Cannabis* plant somewhat for you and that it has helped shed some light on some of finer details with regard to both marijuana and hemp as they relate back to the topic of cannabis oils.

*Cannabis* is an incredibly complex plant, and it is often frustrating to see it reduced into overly simplified terms such as THC content or CBD concentration. Many assumptions are made about cannabis when we still have so much to learn about the vast array of substances contained within the plants.

For 50 years, our culture has focused on one cannabinoid in the cannabis plant: THC. The last decade has seen the focus shift to CBD, and the results of this shift have been dramatic. Who knows what the next decade will bring, with some 100 other cannabinoids yet to be studied!

Cannabis is a very personal substance, reacting within each of us in differing ways. By exploring some of the intricacies of marijuana and hemp, one reaches a higher understanding of the overall potential that plants from the *Cannabis* genus offer us all.

It is my hope that armed with the basic information contained within this book, you will now be able to make some informed judgments with regard to cannabis and cannabis oils, and that this information will benefit you in the future should you decide to either experiment with or purchase cannabis oil. I have tried to present the basic information I feel is important without drowning you in data in the process, and I encourage further study into any specific areas that particularly interest you.

I sincerely hope that this book will aid you in reaching a deeper understanding of the plant and help illustrate how to incorporate various cannabis and cannabis oils into your life to address the specific concerns that might have led you to reading this book in the first place. I wish you the best of health moving forward!

# About the Author

Douglas McCort is a passionate advocate for the medicinal use of cannabis and is a firm believer in the use and value of natural plant-based substances as a substitute for the often harmful alternatives offered up by Big Pharma. He feels strongly that cannabis should be viewed as a tool for life enhancement and healing, and not viewed as an intoxicant. He also chooses to live his life free from alcohol, drugs, and synthetic pharmaceuticals.

Douglas has lived with cyclical vomiting syndrome for the better part of 40 years and feels that cannabis has been one of the only effective tools for dealing with this illness in a healthy and productive way, when most pharmaceuticals he has been given have proven to be either ineffective or harmful. Doug began his medicinal use of cannabis as a late teenager when he discovered it helped cure his lifelong insomnia, in particular. He has used cannabis for medicinal purposes to battle his debilitating nausea and vomiting as well as recreational enhancement for some three decades now.

Douglas has been doing independent research on cannabis for 30 years. He has a lifelong interest and passion for learning about plant-based substances and pharmaceuticals as well as their effects on the body, having purchased his first physician's desk reference guide at the age of 16 after becoming alarmed at some of the pharmaceuticals that were being prescribed to treat his chronic stomach problems.

In addition to his passion for all things cannabis, Douglas has a degree in audio engineering, and is a musician, artist, carpenter, electrician, painter, mechanic, Webmaster, PC gamer, and animal lover. He currently runs a couple of informational blogs regarding hemp-based cannabis oils at cannabisoilforsale.net and cbdmarijuanaoil.com and also runs his own Internet marketing company.

Doug currently resides in his hometown of North Pole, Alaska.

www.ingramcontent.com/pod-product-compliance
Lightning Source LLC
Chambersburg PA
CBHW072212280526
45788CB00002B/982